SJ
ALLE ZEIT WACH
1842

H.G. Hansen E. Graucob

# Hematologic Cytology of Storage Diseases

With 181 Figures, 172 in Colour

Springer-Verlag
Berlin Heidelberg NewYork Tokyo

Professor Dr. Hans Georg Hansen
Elisabeth Graucob
Medizinische Hochschule Lübeck
Klinik für Pädiatrie
Kahlhorststraße 31–35
2400 Lübeck 1

*Printed with the support of the "Förderungs- und Beihilfefonds Wissenschaft der VG Wort"*

Translated into English by Dr. Helen K. Cooper-Schlüter, Aachen,
Title of the German original edition:
Hämatologische Zytologie der Speicherkrankheiten.

ISBN-13: 978-3-642-70059-0 e-ISBN: 978-3-642-70057-6
DOI: 10.1007/978-3-642-70057-6

Library of Congress Cataloging in Publication Data
Hansen, Hans Georg.
Hematologic cytology of storage diseases.
Translation of: Hämatologische Zytologie der Speicherkrankheiten.
Bibliography: p. Includes index.
1. Lysosomal storage diseases – Diagnosis. 2. Blood cells – Examination. 3. Diagnosis, Cytologic. I. Graucob, E. (Elisabeth), 1935– . II. Title. [DNLM: 1. Cystinosis – blood. 2. Glycogenosis – blood. 3. Mucolipidosis – blood. 4. Mucopolysaccharidosis – blood. 5. Sphingolipidosis – blood. WD 205 H249h]
RC632.L94H3613 1985 616.3'995 84-28601


Softcover reprint of the hardcover 1st Edition 1985



2123/3140-543210

# Contents

# Introduction

Das ist das Schwerste von allem,
was Dir das Leichteste dünket:
mit den Augen zu sehen,
was vor den Augen Dir liegt.
Goethe, Xenien, 1797

That is the most difficult
which seems the easiest:
to see with your eyes
what lies there to be seen.

All the diseases in question here are rare. The most common, mucopolysaccharidosis (MPSosis III), occurs at a rate of 1 in 160000. Consequently, any one doctor will only encounter a few cases as a rule, and the literature offers mainly casuistic descriptions. Up till now, there has been no systematic and comprehensive review. We thus felt that it would be of interest and benefit to prepare a collective report on a large body of material gathered over a period of many years, the material being extensive enough to provide adequate possibilities for making comparisons. In so doing, we were also able to describe for the first time the specific, and, in some cases, the pathognomonic symptoms for each disease.

In the past, the nomenclature of these disorders has been changed several times. Originally, the so-called classic storage diseases such as Gaucher's disease, Niemann-Pick disease, and amaurotic idiocy were defined solely from a clinical point of view. For a long time, the terms amaurotic idiocy and dysostosis multiplex included quite different diseases. The first significant progress in the field was the demonstration by Dorfman and Lorincz [8] in 1957 of the increased excretion of acid mucopolysaccharides (aMPS) in the urine of MPSosis patients. As a result, it was possible to characterize six different forms of MPSoses. Furthermore, it was possible to distinguish the large group of mucolipidoses (MLoses) by the absence of mucopolysachariduria (MPSuria). About a decade later, an important step in the further characterization was the recognition that in these forms of inborn errors of metabolism, degradation rather than synthesis is impaired; this was demonstrated in fibroblast cultures [12]. Many enzyme defects were thereafter detected in rapid succession, the first being the defect underlying Austin's disease, described in 1965 [2]. Today, the enzyme defect in most of the diseases in question is known (Tables 1 and 2, see pp. 6–9).

In the majority of cases, one enzyme is either absent or deficient. Occasionally, however, two isoenzymes are affected, probably owing to defects in protein chains common to both. For example, in Austin's disease, arylsulfatases A and B are deficient. The situation in MLosis II and III is quite different. In these cases there is a disturbance not in the synthesis but in the transport of multiple lysosomal enzymes, i.e., they do not reach the site of their action. As a result, enzyme deficiencies in the lysosome ensue, accompanied by high serum levels. The reason is a defective *N*-acetyl-glucosaminyl-phosphotransferase [45].

A remarkable and hitherto inexplicable phenomenon is that one and the same enzyme defect leads to two quite different clinical pictures in the case of MPSosis I–H and I–S, whereas in an apparently uniform clinical picture, as in the case of MPSosis III, at least three different basic defects are known.

The nomenclature used at present is derived from the substance stored, the enzyme defect, or the authors who first described the condition. Biochemically, in the MPSoses and MLoses (heteroglycanoses), as well as in the sphingolipidoses, the degradation of carbohydrate complexes (glycosaminoglycans, glycoproteins, glycosphingolipids) is impaired. Normally, these complex carbohydrates are degraded by a large number of lysosomal enzymes. Should one or more of the enzymes be absent, or be present only in a reduced concentration, metabolites will accumulate in the lysosomes. This intracellular storage is often cytomorphologically (more or less) recognizable. According to the substance stored and the cell system mainly, either mesenchymal (especially skeleton, liver, spleen, and bone marrow) or neurological symptoms predominate clinically. In other words, signs of dysmorphism (e.g., a tendency toward so-called gargoylism) and dysostosis multiplex are clinically prevalent in cases of MPSosis. In contrast, the clinical picture in sphingolipidoses is characterized by a neurological – though variable – syndrome. From both a clinical and a cytomorphological viewpoint, the MLoses occupy a place between the MPSoses and the sphingolipidoses. In this context, we would like to retain the subdivision of the heteroglycanoses into MPSoses and MLoses, since these two groups differ fundamentally in their hematomorphology.

# Clinical Experience

The semiotics of certain clinical pictures, for instance, from the group of MPsoses, have been well known for a long time. This is true for Hunter's syndrome (1917) [21], Pfaundler-Hurler disease (1919) [40, 22], and Morquio's syndrome (1929) [35]. However, these diseases are representative only of the

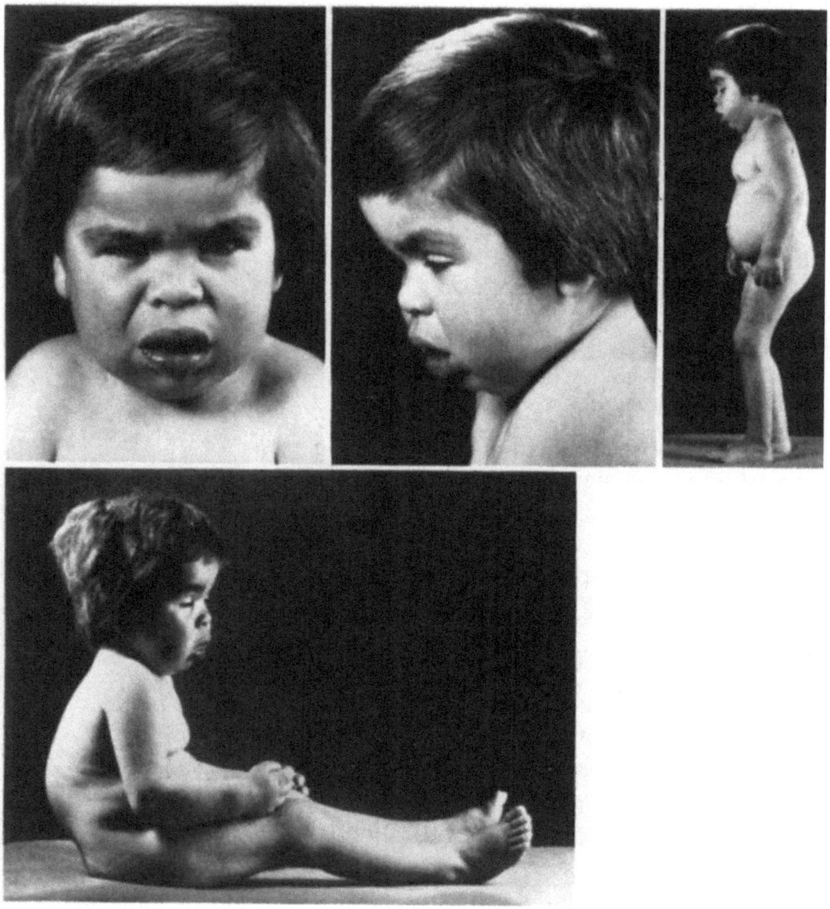

**Fig. 1.** Very typical clinical aspect of mucopolysaccharidosis I–H.

severest forms of a much larger group of similar metabolic defects. Consequently, diagnostic problems do not arise with a child of the phenotype shown in Fig. 1, such a phenotype is highly characteristic of type I–H of the MPSoses, Pfaundler-Hurler disease.

The major symptoms are:

Dysmorphism (gargoyle-like features)
Skeletal changes
Growth retardation
Mental retardation
Corneal clouding
Deafness
Hepatosplenomegaly

However, such a classic phenotype seldom occurs. Although the changes are principly the same in all forms of the disease, they differ remarkably in degree, sometimes even within one type. For this reason, it is important to recognize those minor symptoms which can provide diagnostic guidelines in the early stages of the disease, particularly since these symptoms are relatively constant:

Large head
Saddle nose
Hypertelorism
Hypertrichosis (especially eyebrows)
Macroglossia
Hepatomegaly and/or splenomegaly
Tendency to hernias

Other important indicative symptoms include:

Corneal clouding
Cherry red spot
Impaired hearing

The earliest and most significant radiological signs are:

Hyperostosis of the calvarium
Flat sella turcica
Ovoid or hook-shaped lumbar vertebrae
Upright positioning of acetabula

If these minor clinical symptoms are present and the disease is suspected, laboratory diagnosis is then performed with regard to:

1. Storage phenomena in blood and bone marrow smears
2. In heteroglycanoses: excretion of aMPS or oligosaccharides in urine
3. In lipidoses: suralis biopsy
4. Enzyme diagnosis (leukocytes, serum, fibroblasts)

As can be seen from Tables 1–3, storage phenomena can be demonstrated in the blood and bone marrow in all heteroglycanoses and in most lipidoses. It should be mentioned that this sort of screening is rapid and relatively easy to carry out, providing efficient indications for subsequent biochemical tests.

Furthermore, the hematologic changes can be positively identified before any suspicious clinical sign exists. Thus, for example, we were able to demonstrate storage phenomena in the blood cells of a 6-week-old infant with MPSosis I–H and an 8-month-old girl suffering from mannosidosis.

**Table 1.** Conspectus of age at manifestation, clinical symptoms, and diagnostics in mucopolysaccharidoses

| Name | Synonym | Age at manifestation (year) | Clinical symptoms[a] | | | |
|---|---|---|---|---|---|---|
| | | | Skeletal dysplasia | Dysmorphism | Mental retardation | Corneal clouding |
| MPSosis I–H | Pfaundler-Hurler disease | 1st | + + + | + + + | + + | + (early) |
| MPSosis I–S | Scheie's disease | > 6th | + | (+) | ∅ | + |
| MPSosis I–H/S | "Compound" | > 2nd | + + | + + | + | + |
| MPSosis II A | Hunter's syndrome A | > 2nd | + + + | + + + | + | usually ∅ |
| MPSosis II B | Hunter's syndrome B | > 2nd | + + | + | ∅ | usually ∅ |
| MPSosis III A | Sanfilippo's syndrome A | > 2nd | + | + | + + + | ∅ |
| MPSosis III B | Sanfilippo's syndrome B | > 2nd | + | + | + + + | ∅ |
| MPSosis IV | Morquio's syndrome | > 1st | + + + (spondylo-epiphyseal) | ∅ | ∅ | (+) |
| MPSosis VI | Maroteaux-Lamy syndrome | A > 3rd<br>B > 6th | + + to + + + | + to + + + | ∅ | + |
| MPSosis VII | β-Glucuronidase-deficiency | > 3rd | + to + + | + to + + | ∅ to + | ∅ |

[a] + to + + +, range of clinical expression from slight to very marked

| Urinary excretion (aMPSuria) | Enzyme defect | Detectable in | | | Storage cells | |
|---|---|---|---|---|---|---|
| | | Serum | Leuko-cytes | Fibro-blasts | Blood | Bone marrow |
| Dermatan sulfate<br>Heparan sulfate | α-L-Iduronidase | | + | + | + | + |
| Dermatan sulfate | α-L-Iduronidase | | + | + | + | + |
| Dermatan sulfate<br>Heparan sulfate | α-L-Iduronidase | | + | + | + | + |
| Heparan sulfate<br>Dermatan sulfate | Sulfoiduronate sulfatase | + | + | + | + | + |
| Heparan sulfate<br>Dermatan sulfate | Sulfoiduronate sulfatase | + | + | + | + | + |
| Heparan sulfate | Heparan sulfate sulfamidase | | + | + | + | + |
| Heparan sulfate | *N*-Acetyl-α-D-glucosaminidase | + | + | + | + | + |
| Keratan sulfate<br>Chondroitin sulfate | Galactosamine-6-sulfate-sulfatase | | | + | + | + |
| Dermatan sulfate | Arylsulfatase B = Galactosamine-4-sulfate-sulfatase | | + | + | + | + |
| Dermatan sulfate<br>Heparan sulfate | β-Glucuronidase | + | + | + | + | + |

**Table 2.** Conspectus of semiology and diagnostics of mucolipidoses

| Name | Synonym | Age at manifestation (year) | Clinical symptoms | | | |
|---|---|---|---|---|---|---|
| | | | Skeletal dysplasia | Dysmorphism | Mental retardation | Corneal clouding |
| β-Galactosidase deficiency I | $G_{M1}$-gangliosidosis I | 1st | +++ | +++ | ++ | ∅ (cherry red spot) (50%) |
| β-Galactosidase deficiency II | $G_{M1}$-gangliosidosis II | 2nd | (+) | (+) | + | ∅ |
| β-Galactosidase deficiency III | | 4th to 8th | ++ (spondylo-epiphyseal) | ∅ | ∅ to + | + |
| Fucosidosis I | | 1st | (+) | (+) | +++ | ∅ |
| Fucosidosis II | | 2nd | ++ (spondylo-epiphyseal) | ++ | ++ | + |
| Mannosidosis | | >2nd | + | + | ++ | ∅ |
| Aspartyl-glucosaminuria | | >4th | + | + | ++ | ∅ |
| Mucosulfatidosis | Austin's disease | 2nd | + | (+) | +++ | ∅ |
| Mucolipidosis I | Sialidosis | >2nd | + | + | ++ | ∅ (cherry red spot) |
| Mucolipidosis II | I-cell disease | 1st | +++ | +++ | +++ | + |
| Mucolipidosis III | Pseudo-polydystrophy | >1st | + to +++ | + to +++ | ∅ to +++ | + |

See Table 1 for definition of + to +++

| Urinary excretion | Enzyme defect | Detectable in | | | Storage cells | |
|---|---|---|---|---|---|---|
| | | Serum | Leuko-cytes | Fibro-blasts | Blood | Bone marrow |
| Oligosaccharides Keratan sulfate | β-D-Galactosidase | + | + | + | + | + |
| Oligosaccharides Keratan sulfate | β-D-Galactosidase | + | + | + | + | + |
| Oligosaccharides Keratan sulfate | β-D-Galactosidase | + | + | + | + | + |
| Fucose-containing oligosaccharides | α-L-Fucosidase | | + | + | + | + |
| Fucose-containing oligosaccharides | α-L-Fucosidase | | + | + | + | + |
| Mannose-containing oligosaccharides | α-D-Mannosidase | + | + | + | + | + |
| Aspartyl-glucosamine | Aspartylglucosaminidase | + | + | + | + | ? |
| Dermatan sulfate Heparan sulfate Sulfatid | Arylsulfatases A and B | + (A) | + | + | + | + |
| Neuraminic acid-containing oligosaccharides | α-Neuraminidase | | | + | + | + |
| | *N*-Acetylglucosaminyl-phosphotransferase | | + | + | + | + |
| | *N*-Acetylglucosaminyl-phosphotransferase | | + | + | ∅ and + | ∅ and + |

**Table 3.** Conspectus of age at manifestation, clinical symptoms, and enzyme defects in lipidoses

| Name | Synonym | Age at manifestation | Clinical symptoms | | | Enzyme defect | Detectable in | | | Storage cells | |
|---|---|---|---|---|---|---|---|---|---|---|---|
| | | | Viscera | Neurological symptoms | Eyes (cherry red spot) | | Serum | Leukocytes | Fibroblasts | Blood | Bone marrow |
| **Niemann-Pick disease** | | | | | | | | | | | |
| Type A | | > 3rd month | + + | + | + (50%) clouding of lenses | Sphingomyelinase | | | + | ? | + |
| Type B | | > 2nd year | + + + | ∅ | ∅ | Sphingomyelinase | | | + | | + |
| Type C | | > 2nd year | + | + + | + | Sphingomyelinase, partial defect | | | + | ∅ | + |
| Type D | "Nova Scotia" variant | > 5th year | + | + + | ∅ | Sphingomyelinase, partial defect | | | + | | + |
| Type E | | | + + | ∅ | ∅ | Sphingomyelinase, partial defect | | | + | | + |
| Type F | „Sea-blue histiocyte disease“ | > 4th year | + + | ∅ to + + | ∅ | thermolabile sphingomyelinase | | | + | ∅ | + |
| **Krabbe's disease** | | | | | | | | | | | |
| Late infantile | Globoid cell leukodystrophy | > 3rd month | ∅ | + + + | ∅ Optic atrophy | Galactocerebroside-β-galaktosidase | | + | + | ∅ | ∅ |
| Juvenile | | > 3rd year | ∅ | + + | ∅ | Galactocerebroside-β-galaktosidase | | + | + | ∅ | ∅ |
| Adult | | > 5th year | ∅ | + | ∅ | Galactocerebroside-β-galaktosidase | | + | + | ∅ | ∅ |

| | | | | | | | | | | | |
|---|---|---|---|---|---|---|---|---|---|---|---|
| **Metachromatic leukodystrophy** | | | | | | | | | | | |
| Late infantile | | >9th month | Ø | +++ | Ø Optic atrophy | Arylsulfatase A | + | + | + | Ø | Ø |
| Juvenile | | >5th year | Ø | ++ | Ø | Arylsulfatase A | + | + | + | Ø | Ø |
| Adult | | >10th year | Ø | + | Ø | Arylsulfatase A | + | + | + | Ø | Ø |
| **Gaucher's disease** | | | | | | | | | | | |
| Infantile | | >3rd month | ++ | ++ | Ø (rare) | Glucocerebroside-β-glucosidase | | + | + | Ø | + |
| Juvenile | | >1st year | +++ | + | Ø | Glucocerebroside-β-glucosidase | | + | + | Ø | + |
| Adult | | 1st year | +++ | Ø to (+) | Ø | Glucocerebroside-β-glucosidase | | + | + | Ø | + |
| **Fabry's disease** | | | | | | | | | | | |
| | Angiokeratoma corporis diffusum universale | >5th year | vessels | Ø | Ø clouding of lenses | α-Galactosidase | + (Plasma) | + | + | Ø | Ø |
| **$G_{M2}$-Gangliosidoses** | | | | | | | | | | | |
| Type I | Tay-Sachs disease | <6th month | Ø | ++ | + | β-Hexosaminidase A | + | + | + | Ø | + |
| Type II | Bernheimer-Seitelberger disease | >6th month | Ø | ++ | + (50%) | β-Hexosaminidase A | + | + | + | Ø | ? |
| Type III | Sandhoff's disease | <6th month | + | ++ | + (50%) | β-Hexosaminidase A and B | + | + | + | Ø | (+) |

See Table 1 for definition of + to +++

# Preliminary Remarks Concerning Cytology

## Material, Methods and Techniques

### *Material*

The data presented here are based on blood and bone marrow studies performed on a series of patients, most of whom were diagnosed and followed up by SPRANGER (Mainz). Other valuable preparations were contributed by DI FERRANTE (Houston), MAROTEAUX (Paris), MAUMENEE and MCKUSICK (Baltimore), OPITZ (Madison), RAMPINI (Zürich), WIEDEMANN (Kiel), and others (see page 71). Only through this successful international cooperation, reinforced by an international therapy program and cytological follow-ups, was it possible to obtain a comparatively large amount of material (Table 4). With such rare diseases, it is not surprising that a few omissions remain. In addition, we had preparations from patients apparently suffering from exceedingly rare and as yet unidentified diseases (see "other forms"). Those patients whose cytological findings cannot be clearly associated with any of the defined diseases are included in the group "unclassified."

In general, the bone marrow and blood smears examined had been sent unstained, unfixed, and air-dried. Conventional smear preparations were preferred to so-called coverslips. The latter have proved unsuitable because storage cells often tend to cluster in certain regions and it is not unusual for these cells to be more or less artificially damaged. Moreover, these preparations are sometimes too thick or more particularly too closely packed.

It is generally desirable to examine both blood *and* bone marrow, although for the diagnosis of some forms (e.g., MLosis II, MPSosis III) a blood smear, and for other forms (e.g., $G_{M1}$-gangliosidosis II, lipidoses) a bone marrow sample suffice.

In assessing the findings, the age of the patients should be taken into account to some extent. For, although it is by no means the case that the oldest patients always have the most pronounced cytological changes, storage phenomena are nonetheless relatively slight in youngest patients. Preparations taken from children of different ages suggest that the extent of storage increases during the first few years of life, however this is not evident after about 5 years of age. In a few patients we were able to observe the course of the disease over a period of up to 5 years; repeated examinations of these children showed that there was no significant increase in storage.

**Table 4.** Classification of the 229 cases of storage diseases included in study

| Heteroglycanoses | | | | Lipidoses | |
|---|---|---|---|---|---|
| Mucopolysaccharidoses | Patients (*n*) | Mucolipidoses | Patients (*n*) | | Patients (*n*) |
| MPSosis | | β-Galactosidase deficiency type I | 5 | Niemann-Pick disease | 3 |
| I–H (Hurler's disease) | 23 | β-Galactosidase deficiency type II und III | 6 | "Sea-blue histiocyte disease" | 7 |
| I–S (Scheie's disease) | 5 | Fucosidosis | 1 | Krabbe's disease | – |
| I–H/S ("Compound") | 7 | Mannosidosis | 18 | Metachromatic leukodystrophy | 1 |
| II (Hunter's syndrome) | 31 | Aspartyl-glucosaminuria | 2 | Gaucher's disease | 4 |
| III (Sanfilippo's syndrome) | 35 | Mucosulfatidosis (Austin) | 5 | Fabry's disease | – |
| IV (Morquio's syndrome) | 13 | Mucolipidosis I (Sialidosis) | 2 | Tay-Sachs disease | 2 |
| VI (Maroteaux-Lamy syndrome | 13 | Mucolipidosis II (I-cell disease) | 13 | Sandhoff's disease | 3 |
| VII (β-Glucuronidase deficiency) | 4 | Mukolipidosis III (Pseudo-polydystrophy) | 10 | Ceroidlipofuscinosis | 4 |
| Other forms | 1 | Unclassified | 6 | | |
| Unclassified | 5 | | | | |
| | 137 | | 68 | | 24 |

## *Methods and Techniques*

All preparations were stained with the May-Grünwald-Giemsa reagents, which are very stable, easy to use and reproducible. For many years we also employed toluidine blue staining regularly and to some extent examined experimentally many technical modifications. The results showed that while toluidine blue is certainly an attractive dye, the results obtained with it depend a great deal on the permanent good quality of the stain, which is by no means always assured. Moreover, the pH or the kind of solvents can affect the results. Thus, toluidine blue staining proved unsatisfactory for this purpose. The depiction of specific granules can be improved by the use of a blue filter (according to Di Ferrante). This method was later employed only where specifically indicated. The same is true of alcian blue, PAS, and the acid phosphatase reaction, as well as of various fat-staining methods; however, they were not helpful in providing further guidelines.

With some practice, it is not difficult to differentiate between normal and pathologic cell structures in May-Grünwald-Giemsa samples. In neutrophilic granulocytes, the pathologic granules are not only coarser but are also very irregularly distributed among the normal granules. The same is true for monocytes. In lymphocytes, the normal, fine, azure granulation can easily be distinguished. Difficulties may arise with reactive forms, under certain conditions they can contain relatively coarse granules, too. Substantial granulation is also well known in individuals with leukemia or who are undergoing cytostatic therapy. Vacuoles in lymphocytes can also very rarely occur normally, either at a very low rate – namely, one or two, or at the most, three fine vacuoles per cell – or they are numerous, very fine, and, in contrast to pathologic vacuoles, lined up like pearls on a string below the plasma wall. The morula-like vacuolation typically found in MLoses never occurs in healthy individuals.

As far as possible, all preparations were quantitatively evaluated (see Tables 5–8, Appendix) in order to obtain a general view and to establish possible differences between each form of the various diseases. It should of course be mentioned that the different smear techniques could implicate considerable sources of error. The evaluation is given not only in terms of the percentage of affected cells per cell type; the number per cell and the size of the storage products were also taken into account. The sizes are defined as follows:

| | | |
|---|---|---|
| Granules: | fine | up to 0.5 μm |
| | coarse | 0.5–1.0 μm |
| | lumpy | >1.0 μm |
| Vacuoles: | fine | up to 2.0 μm |
| | coarse | >2.0 μm |

Only as a result of these procedures it gradually became apparent that some criteria for differentiation could be deduced from the data. For example, there is a more pronounced storage in plasma cells in MPSosis II than in MPSosis I–H.

Unless stated otherwise, the changes of the neutrophils, eosinophils, and monocytes in bone marrow correspond to those of the peripheral blood cells. This is completely different in the case of lymphocytes: the well-known uniform and small bone marrow lymphocytes, with apparent absence of cytoplasm, show markedly less storage (probably since they are stem cells with resting metabolism and therefore exhibit no or only a low tendency to storage).

The MPSoses represent a relatively uniform group since storage is always granular and the same cell types are affected in each disease, although at different focal points (see "marker cells" depicted in Fig. 25). We have tried to compare the quantitative findings derived from the MLoses as well. However, it is certain that for the MLoses the marker cells characteristic of each disease are of much more importance (see Fig. 43), and the same is true of the lipidoses.

One preliminary remark is necessary with regard to certain qualitative changes. Today, it is still not uncommon to encounter historical terms such as Alder's or Reilly's granulation. Both authors reported in a merely descriptive manner on these storage phenomena without at that time ascribing them to particular diseases. In 1939, ALDER [1] described a granulation anomaly in all blood leukocytes of two seemingly healthy siblings, one of whom was later reexamined by several specialists. Oddly enough, even today it is not clear what disease the patient is suffering from. We consider it possible to have been a very mild form of β-glucuronidase deficiency. In 1941, REILLY [44] observed that in four out of eight patients suffering from "gargoylism" there was abnormal granulation in some of the granulocytes as well as in some lymphocytes and monocytes. From the descriptions given one can only make an educated guess as to whether the patients had MPSosis I–H. On the other hand, UNDRITZ [60] believed that there was no significant difference between the two types of granulation and designate both as Alder's anomaly. In 1950 GASSER [13] described characteristic inclusions in the blood lymphocytes and reticulum cells of bone marrow in some patients suffering from "gargoylism", and these have subsequently appeared in the literature as Gasser I and Gasser II cells.

Since it is not possible to assign all these morphological changes retrospectively to a certain form of the MPSoses, it does not appear sensible to us to use these historically interesting terms today. The so-called Buhot cell is an exception (see [46]); this bone marrow plasma cell, typified by a multiplicity of polymorphic inclusions, is characteristic of MPSosis III (see Fig. 18).

## Technical Sources of Error

The most common cause of erroneous findings is poor smearing technique. False results can be obtained from bone marrow if there are no small bits of marrow or if these are poorly spread or smeared. Based on our experience, the addition of coagulation inhibitors is not recommended since the cells are thereby more susceptible to damage. This applies also to blood smears. Here, there is the further complication that coagulation inhibitors in native blood can cause morphological changes in the cells even within a short period of time. Also, since aMPS are water-soluble, there is the danger of their dissolving out upon the addition of aqueous solutions such as ethylenediaminetetraacetate (EDTA) or sodium citrate.

Blood and bone marrow preparations should be unfixed, dustfree, and not stored for too long, since aging of the preparation can lead to considerable falsification of the color and to clumping of the granules. Blood smears should not be too thick. At the same time, if they are too thin and smeared under pressure, the storage cells tend to be pushed ahead and become squashed or otherwise severely damaged.

The so-called sandwich technique is not very suitable for this type of investigation because of the imperfect cell dispersion which results (see discussion of coverslips above).

Wright and Giemsa staining should not be used since the pathologic inclusions are less clearly displayed, involving the danger of false-negative results. With Wright staining, the granules are fewer and less distinct; to some extent the granules disappear and are replaced by vacuoles. Localization is thus made more difficult, slight changes are not evident, and marked changes fade away (Fig. 2).

2a 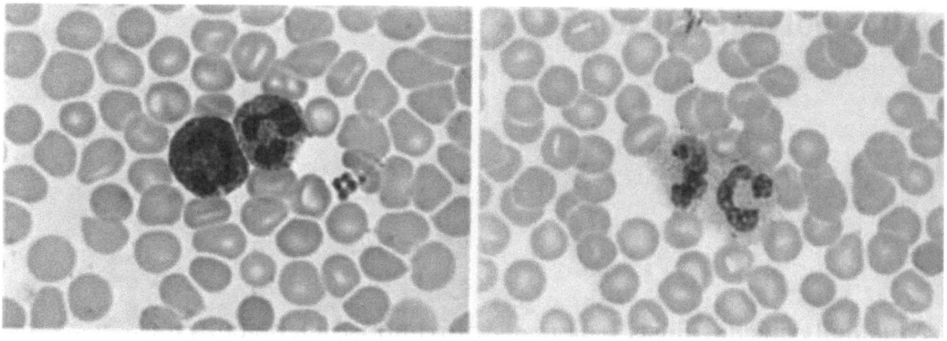 2b

**Fig. 2a, b.** Neutrophilic polymorphs in blood smears from same patient.
**a** May-Grünwald-Giemsa staining: clearly increased granulation.
**b** Wright staining: granules hardly recognizable.

## Cytological Changes in the Different Storage Diseases

The following descriptions are based on the morphology determined with May-Grünwald-Giemsa staining, unless otherwise stated. As a result of alcohol fixation, "halos" or rings of increased translucence around the pathologic granules can occasionally be observed. In our experience, the coarser the granule, the more often they appear.

The frequency data in the text refer to the tables in the Appendix (see pp. 77–83).

---

For the following figures, where not specifically mentioned there is a May-Grünwald-Giemsa stain and a magnification ×800.

# Mucopolysaccharidoses

## Mucopolysaccharidosis I–H ($\alpha$-L-Iduronidase Deficiency) Synonym: Hurler's Disease [22, 40]

In *blood smears* (Figs. 3–6) the neutrophilic granulocytes can show fine, yet quite densly packed granules. More frequently, only sparse inclusions are present. While similar differences are observed in the monocytes, altogether storage here is more pronounced. Likewise, the eosinophils sometimes show discrete storage, i.e., slightly to moderately coarse, greenish granules. Such changes in the granulocytes and monocytes are often found in other MPSoses and are consequently of little importance. The lymphocytes are more significant; the proportion of affected cells differs from patient to patient (43%–90%), and the number of granules varies from cell to cell. They are usually fine and occasionally very densely packed. It is the distribution which is characteristic: the inclusions are for the most part diffusely spread throughout the cytoplasm, a phenomenon that can be observed even in the apparent absence of cytoplasmic seam. If plasma cells are present in the blood smear granules are rarely seen.

**Fig. 3a, b.** MPSosis I–H. Blood. Neutrophilic polymorphs. Slightly coarsened, pathologic granules irregularly scattered throughout the normal granulation.

**Fig. 4.** MPSosis I–H. Blood smear showing eosinophilic granulocytes with slightly coarsened, gray-greenish granulation.

**Fig. 5a, b.** MPSosis I–H. Blood monocytes.
**a** Very fine, very dense, reddish granulation.
**b** Fine, dense granulation and a coarse inclusion with distinct halo.

**Fig. 6a–e.** MPSosis I–H. Blood lymphocytes.
**a, b** Small lymphocytes with very little cytoplasm that is almost completely filled with fine pathologic granules.
**c–d** Lymphocytes with broader cytoplasmic border which contains varying numbers of relatively coarse granules, frequently with a distinct halo.
**e** Storage lymphocytes in the blood of a 6-week-old infant; fortuitous diagnosis as a result of blood finding.

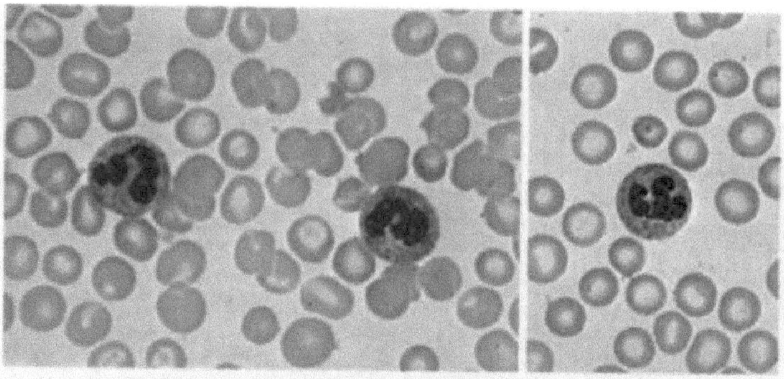
3a, b

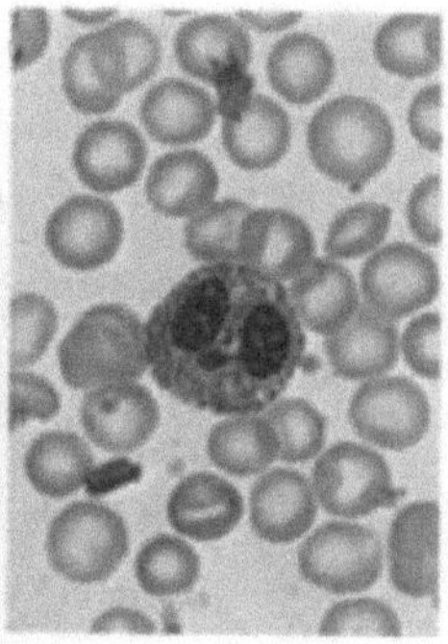
4

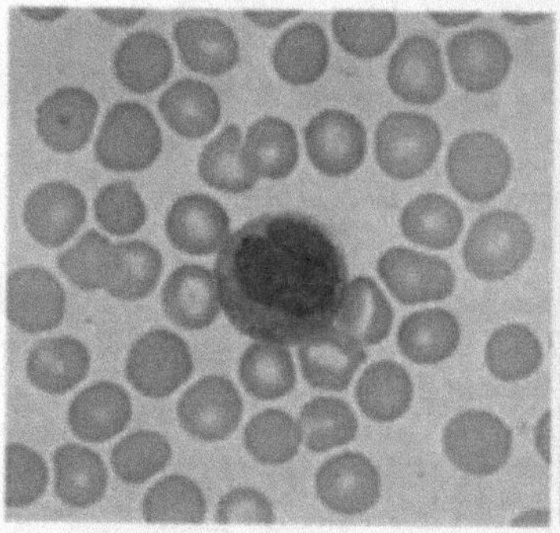
5a

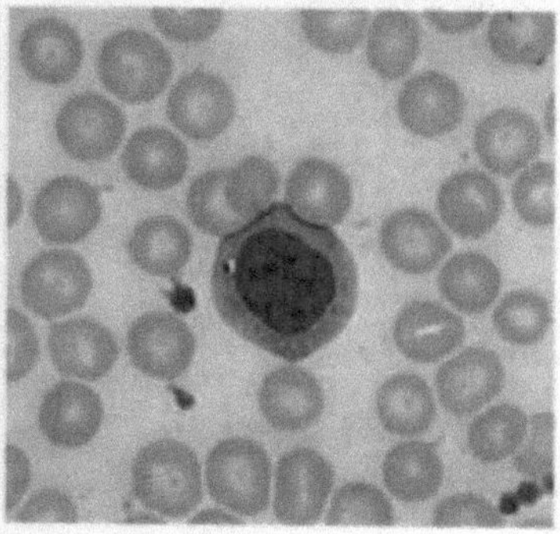
5b

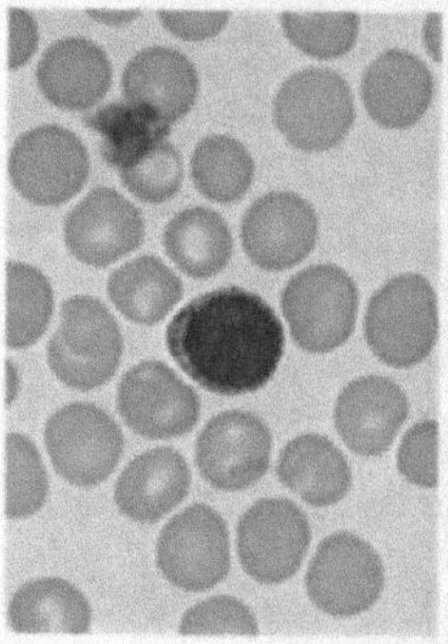
6a

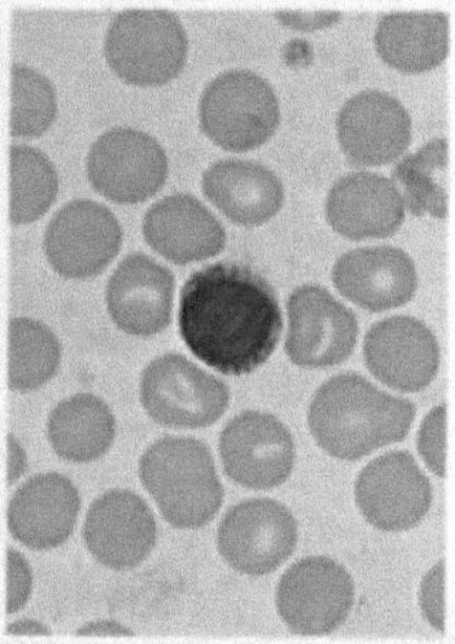
6b

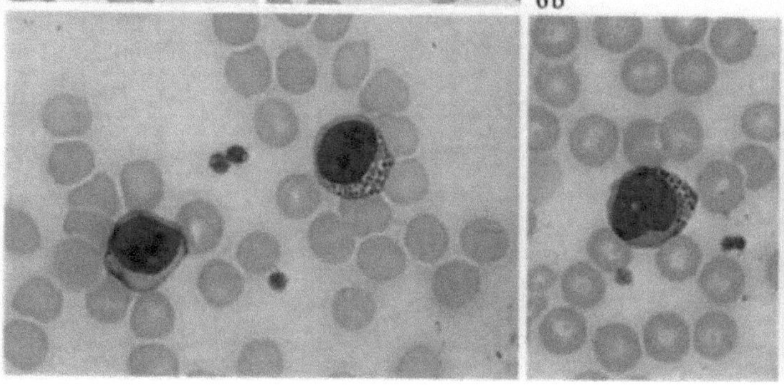
6c, d

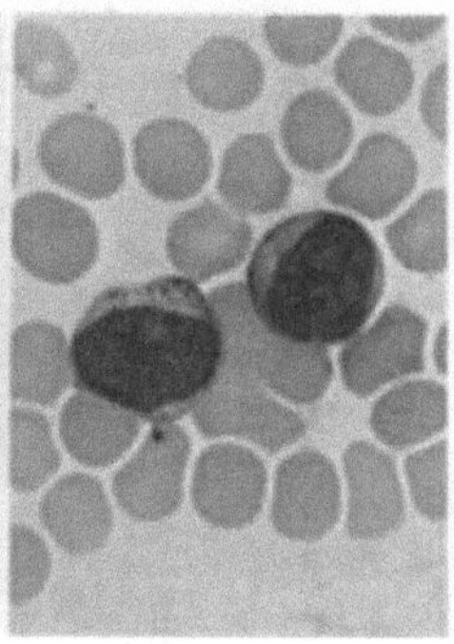
6e

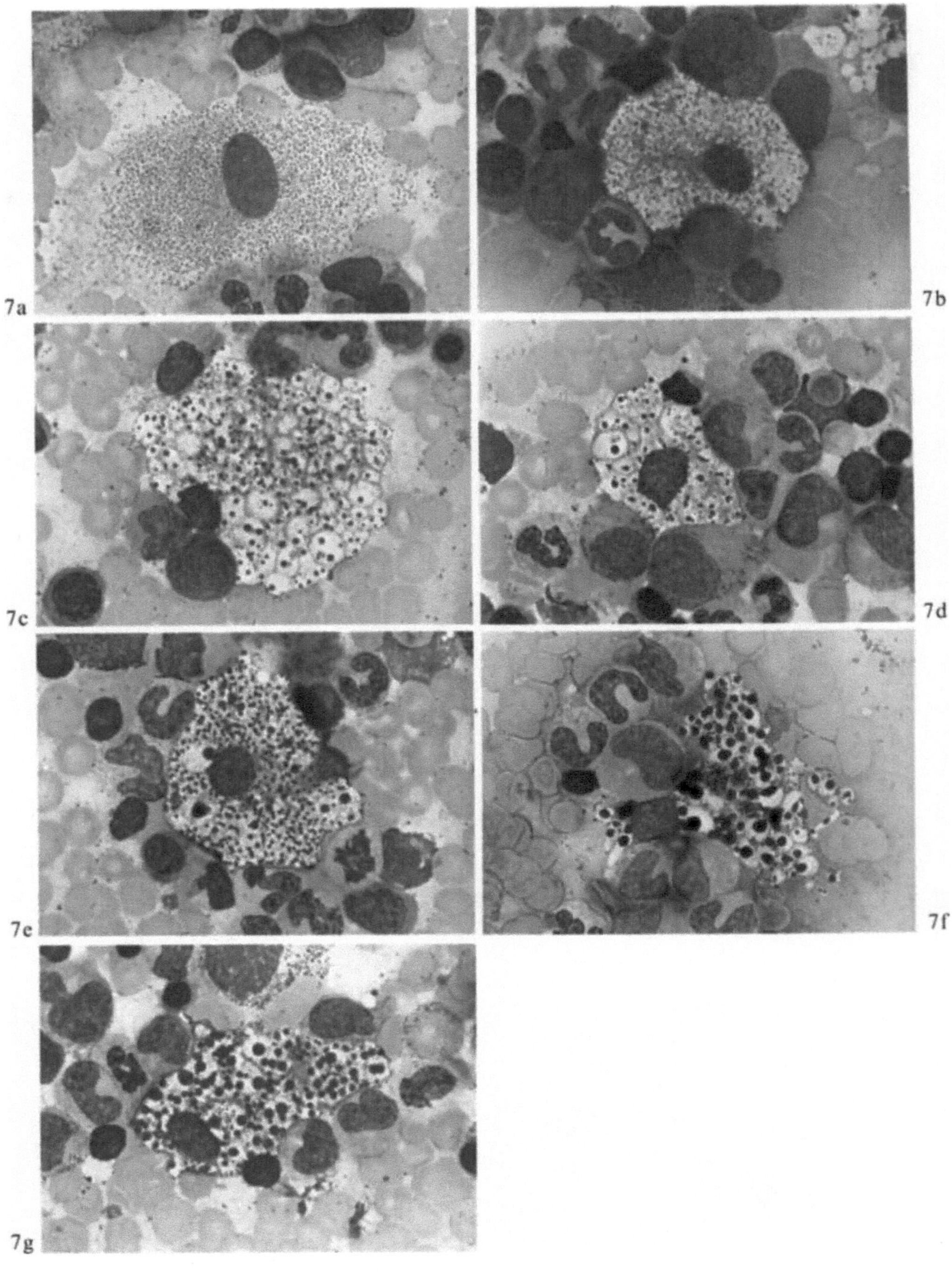


**Fig. 7 a–g.** MPSosis I–H. Reticulum cells in bone marrow. Various forms of storage, from very fine granules to coarse lumps; more or less marked loss of normal, spindly extended cell shape tending to roundish cytoplasm.

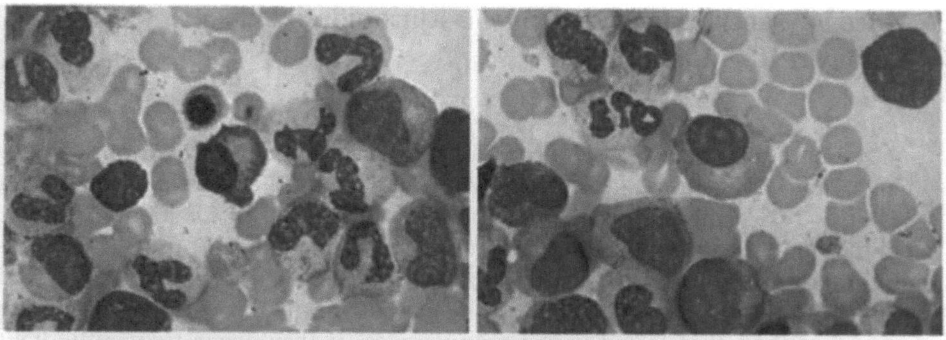

8a

8b

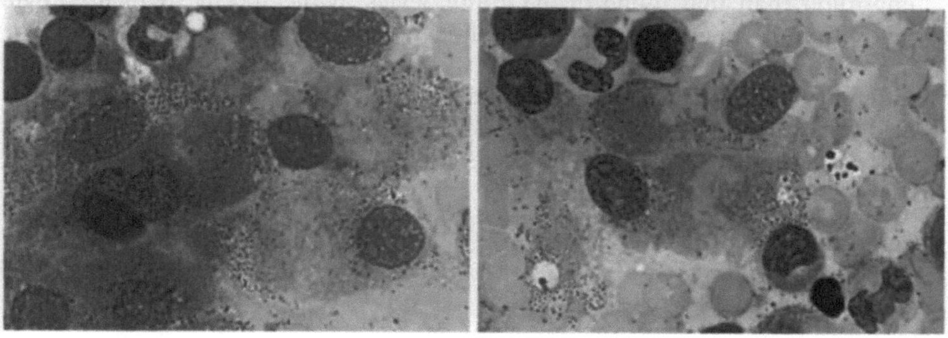

9a

9b

**Fig. 8a, b.** MPSosis I–H. Plasma cells in bone marrow. Only sparse, fine, reddish granules; the cytoplasm is not enlarged.

**Fig. 9a, b.** MPSosis I–H. Osteoblasts in bone marrow. Very numerous, more or less fine granules. The typical cytoplasmic zone of increased translucence remain largely free of granules.

In the *bone marrow,* all reticulum cells exhibit storage phenomena (Fig. 7). However, the inclusions differ with regard to size, number, and shape as well as in distribution. The reticulum cells generally lose their rather spindly, extended form; the cytoplasm is usually enlarged; and sometimes, the nucleus is pyknotic. In MPSosis I–H, in addition to inclusions which are fine or sometimes coarse, granular, uniformly distributed, and dense, there are also *always* inclusions which are lumps of different shapes and sizes and which are as a rule somewhat less numerous and more irregularly distributed (Fig. 7g).

Some of the plasma cells show a few, fine granules (Fig. 8) and occasionally vacuoles. Halos are usually absent. Vacuoles probably correspond to dissolved granules.

Without exception, the osteoblasts, which on close examination are nearly always present in marrow punctates, exhibit considerable granular storage, while the typical cytoplasmic zones of increased translucence remain unfilled (Fig. 9).

In bone marrow preparations there are often free, extracellular, and more or less coarse granules which are clustered together. In our opinion, this storage material originates from damaged reticulohistiocytic elements.

## **Mucopolysaccharidosis I–H/S** (α-L-Iduronidase Deficiency)
Synonym: Compound [33]

The compound type MPSosis I–H/S (a heterogeneous type with various components) and MPSosis II (Hunter's syndrome) cannot be distinguished from MPSosis I–H (Hurler's disease) on the basis of a *blood smear* alone (Fig. 10). On the whole, very marked storage is more consisting with MPSosis I–H, whereas minor storage is more suspective for MPSosis II. In the case of marked storage, it should be added that storage occurring in the monocytes is more important than that found in the granulocytes. If they occur frequently, light halos around the granules in the lymphocytes suggest MPSosis I–H.

*Bone marrow* findings arrived at with panoptical staining are not clearly different. However, when toluidine blue is used in either a neutral or a strongly acidic medium, MPSosis I–H/S produces an intensive metachromasia of the storage substance in the reticulum cells (Fig. 11c, d).

10a 10b

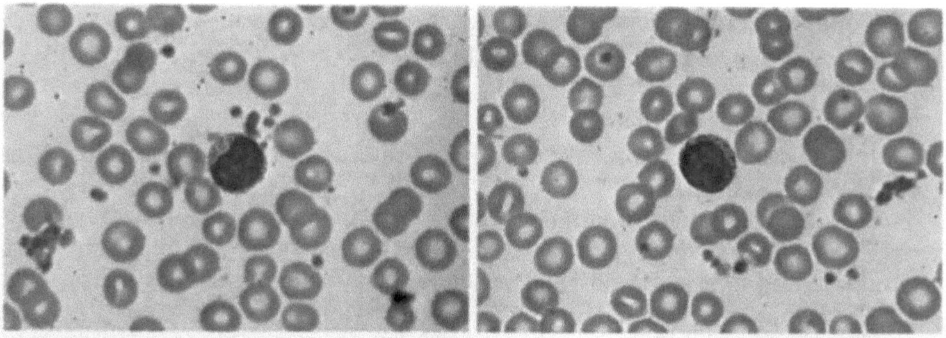

11a 11b
11c 11d

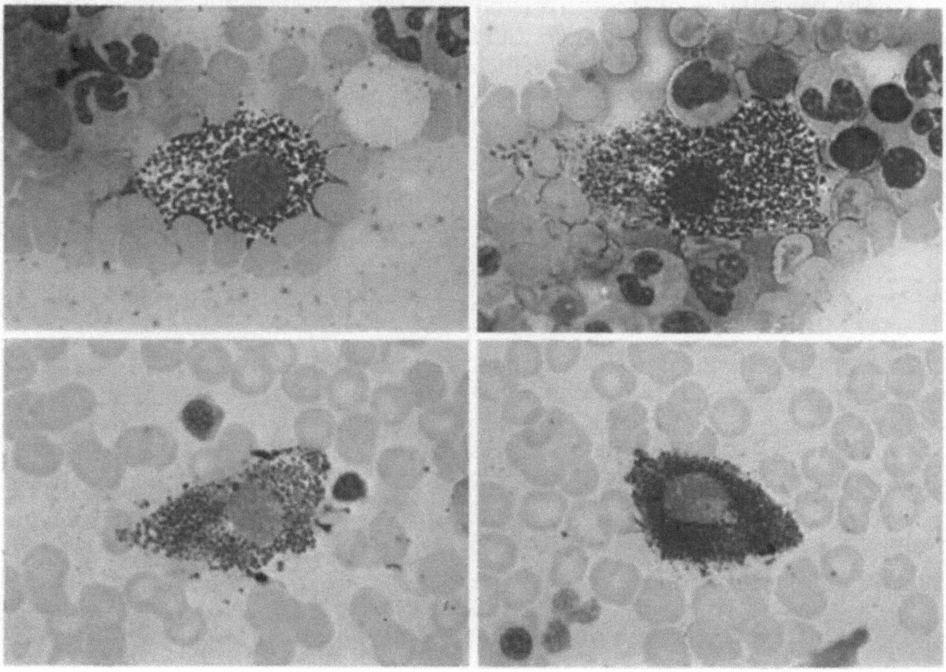

**Fig. 10a, b.** MPSosis I–H/S. Blood lymphocytes. Granular storage visible to varying degrees.

**Fig. 11a–d.** MPSosis I–H/S. Reticulum cells in bone marrow.
**a, b** Very dense, predominantly fine granulation.
**c, d** Toluidine blue staining (pH 3): red-violet metachromasia of pathologic granulation.

**Mucopolysaccharidosis II** (Sulfoiduronate Sulfatase Deficiency)
Synonym: Hunter's Syndrome [21]

With regard to *blood smear,* see the previous section (Mucopolysaccharidosis I–H/S) and Figs. 12 and 13.

Storage phenomena are found in almost all reticulum cells in the *bone marrow*. The storage is predominantly of a fine to coarse granular, regularly dense nature. Lump-like inclusions are present in only some patients (here in four out of seven).

The percentages of storage plasma cells vary considerably (55%–85%), but with one exception, all are none the less higher than those found in Hurler's disease. In MPSosis II as well, the inclusions are predominantly fine and granular but are in part more densely packed, i.e., more numerous (Fig. 14).

The osteoblasts are also always altered, but only on occasion as markedly so as in MPSosis I–H. We also did not find such large amounts of free pigment in MPSosis II.

12
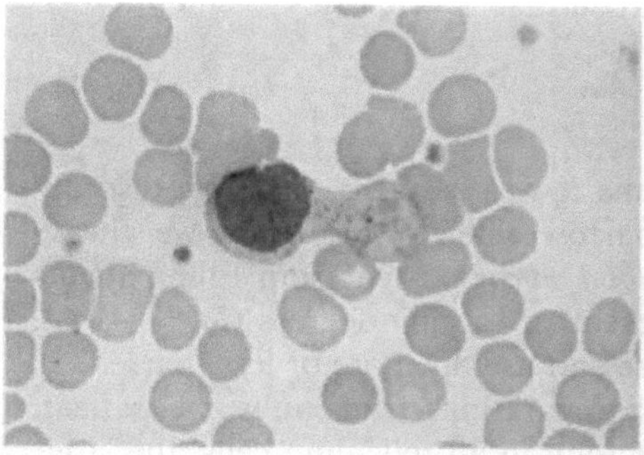
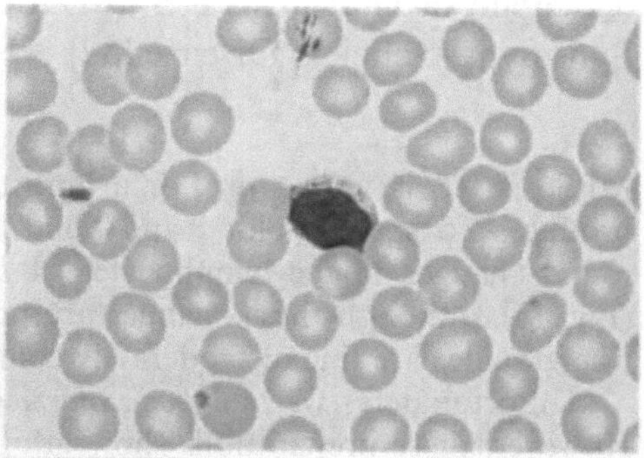
13a

13b
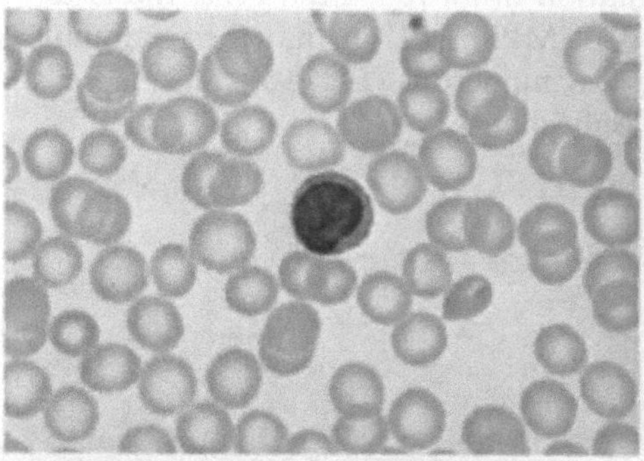
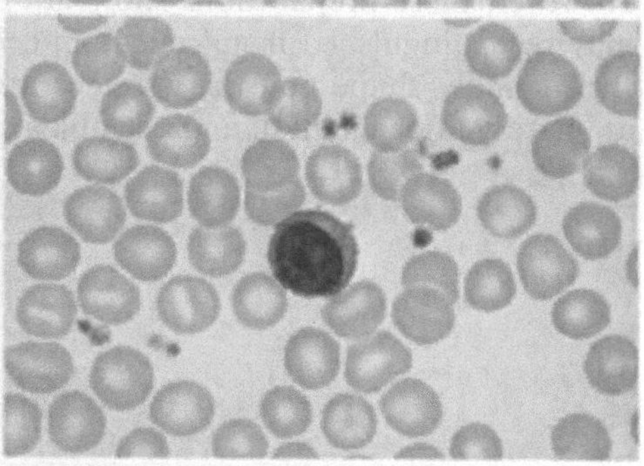
13c

14a
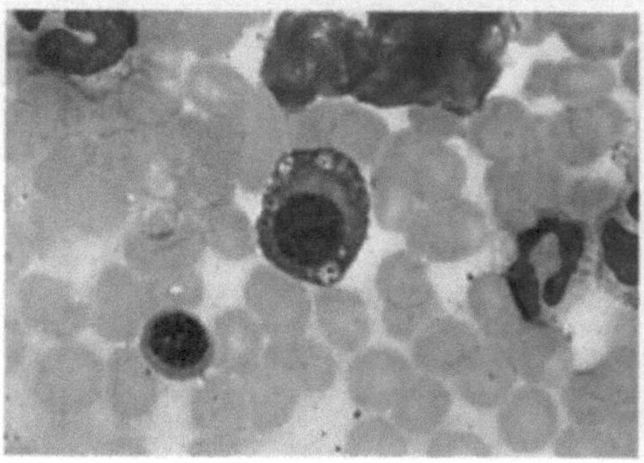
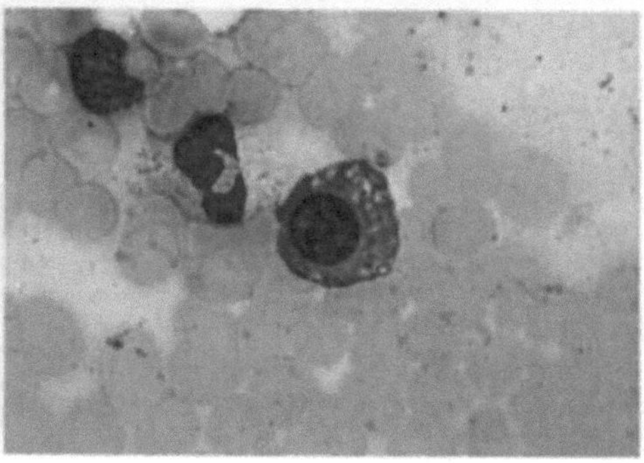
14b

**Fig. 12.** MPSosis II. Blood monocyte with predominantly very fine granular storage.

**Fig. 13a–c.** MPSosis II. Blood lymphocytes. Slight changes with chiefly sparse, fine granules.

**Fig. 14a, b.** MPSosis II. Plasma cells in bone marrow. Relatively numerous, fine and coarse granular, violet inclusions often surrounded by halos.

## **Mucopolysaccharidosis I–S** (α-L-Iduronidase Deficiency)
Synonym: Scheie's Disease [52]

MPSosis I–S is very rare. For a long time it was assumed that this disorder produces no specific blood and bone marrow changes. However, we always found changes in the lymphocytes of *blood smears* taken from four patients (Fig. 15), although these changes are present to varying degrees (3.7%–41%). The granules are fine or moderately coarse and usually more or less sparse.

Unfortunately, we had *bone marrow* preparations from only one patient. However, these preparations show granulation in all reticulum cells, the latter may be distinguished from reticulum cells of MPSosis II in that they maintain their spindly shape and the granules are less numerous (Fig. 16). Plasma cells are hardly affected at all and osteoblasts only slightly.

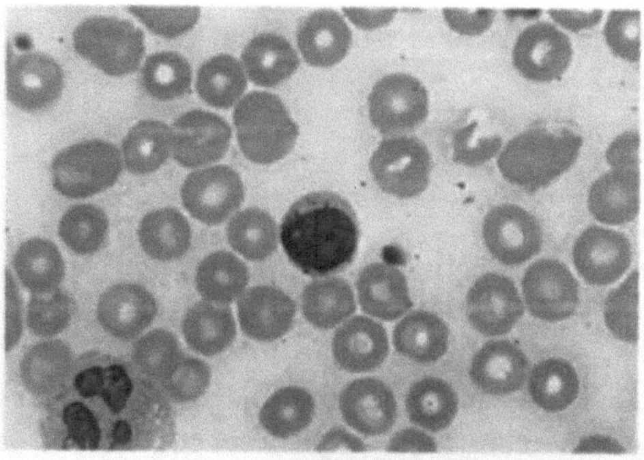

15

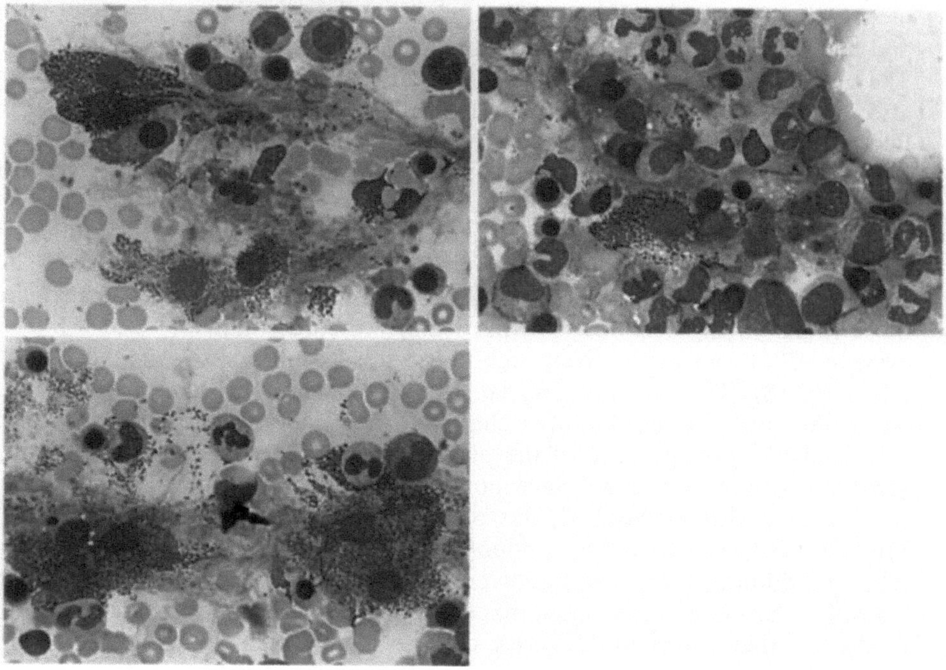

16a

16b

16c

**Fig. 15.** MPSosis I–S. Blood lymphocyte with several fine granules.

**Fig. 16a–c.** MPSosis I–S. Bone marrow. Different degrees of mainly fine granular storage in reticulum cells. The normal spindle shape is usually retained.
**a** Very sparse, fine granules in the plasma cell.
(**a–c** Magnification, × 500).

## **Mucopolysaccharidosis III** (Heparan Sulfate Sulfamidase or *N*-Acetyl-glucosaminidase Deficiency Synonym: Sanfilippo's Syndrome [49]

The morphological findings of the various forms differ as little as their clinical pictures. However, this may be due to the fact that an enzyme analysis was carried out in only nine out of the 35 cases investigated here.

In the *blood smear,* the lymphocytes are the cells to look for. Although the proportion of cells exhibiting granular storage is comparable to that found in MPSosis I–H, I–H/S, and II, the granules are as a rule not only sparser and somewhat coarser but also show a marked tendency to cluster (Fig. 17). The granulation is always restricted to a single plasma area in >50% of the affected lymphocytes. In the remainder, either the granules are distributed in two regions, or there are single, dispersed granules in addition to the clusters. In most cases, halos are rare or absent. A further characteristic is the low proportion of affected granulocytes and monocytes. The changes occurring in MPSosis III are probably those referred to in the literature as the lymphocyte type of Alder's granulation (see [61].

Even more distinctive than the changes described in the blood smear are those found in the *bone marrow,* particularly the quantitatively (75%–100%; average 93%) and qualitatively significant storage phenomena in the plasma cells (Fig. 18). The polymorphic, i.e. rod-, ring-, dumbbell-, or hook-shaped inclusions are extraordinarily characteristic and almost type specific (11.5%–37%; average 23% of the plasma cells). These inclusions are usually surrounded by a large halo. Such polymorphic inclusions were found in only two patients with MPSosis II, out of all those suffering from some form of MPSosis, and even here they amounted to only 1.7% and 2% of the plasma cells. In addition, there are fine or coarse granules, some of which also have halos. Furthermore, it is striking that the cytoplasm is enlarged, i.e., distended.

As in other forms of MPSosis, changes in both the reticulum cells and the osteoblasts are found here, too, but these are considerably less marked than in MPS I–H.

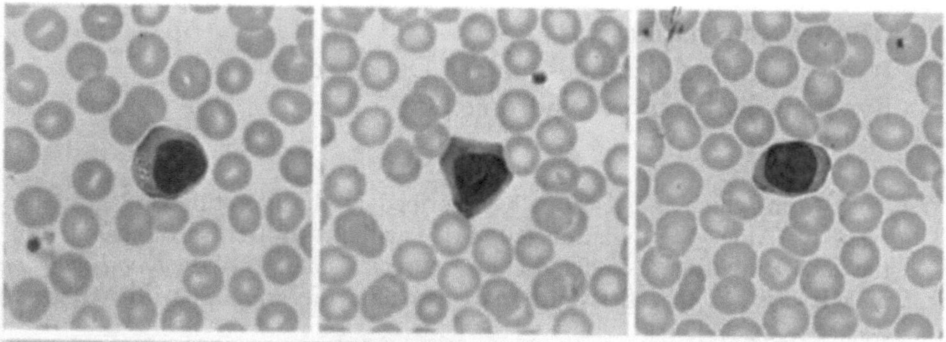

17a, b

17c

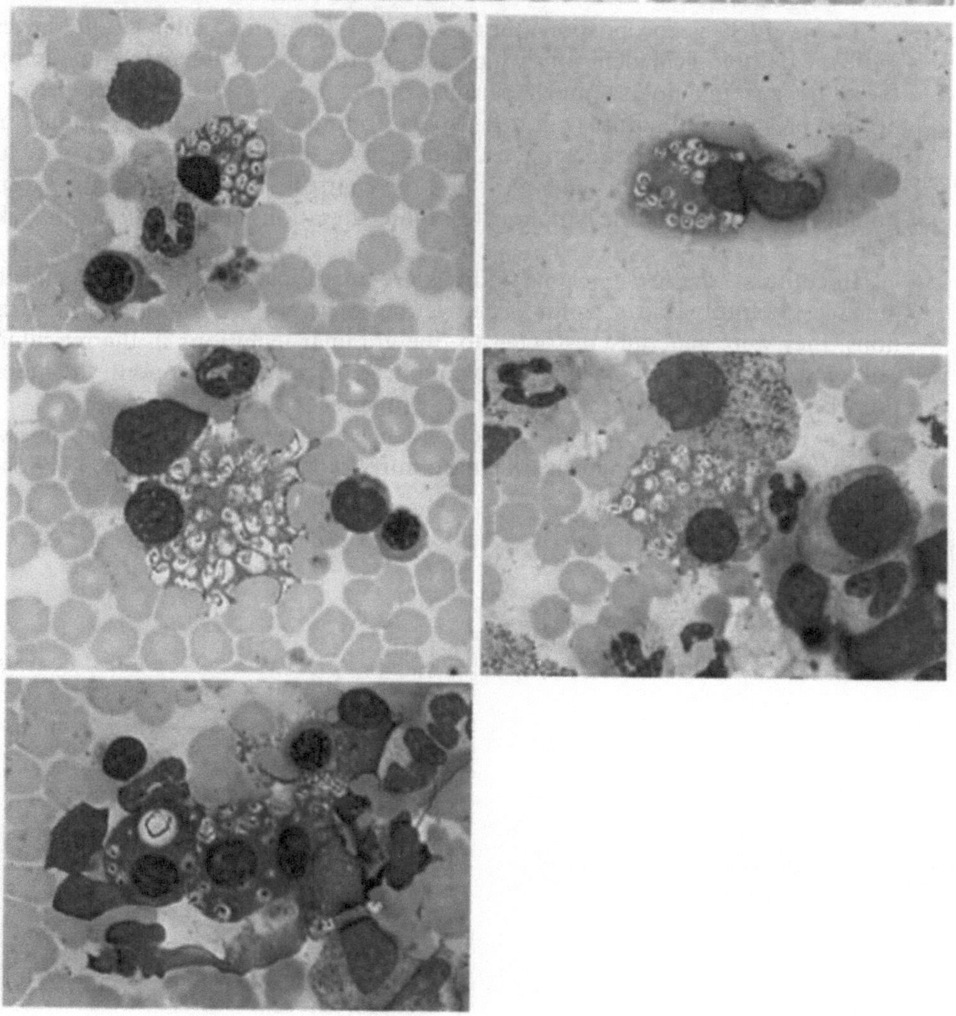

18a

18b

18c

18d

18e

**Fig. 17a–c.** MPSosis III. Blood lymphocytes. Typical clustering of pathologic granules.
**a** Distinct halos.
**c** Two groups of granules.

**Fig. 18a–e.** MPSosis III. Plasma cells in bone marrow. Characteristic, very polymorphic inclusions, surrounded by distinct halos (so-called Buhot cells).

## Mucopolysaccharidosis IV

(Galactosamine-6-sulfatesulfatase Deficiency)
Synonym: Morquio's Syndrome [35]

That form which is occasionally described in the literature as "granulocyte type" of Alder's granulation [10, 61] – without awareness of its relation to the underlying disease – refers to the very typical changes of the *blood neutrophils* in MPSosis IV. The first author to associate the granules with MPSosis IV was McKusick [34].

In a very large proportion (mean 80%) of the neutrophilic granulocytes, there are pathological inclusions which are fine to coarse grained or even lumpy; these are striking not so much because of the number per cell but because of their pronounced nature (Fig. 19). Apart from the classic Alder's granulation in MPSosis VI and VII and mucosulfatidosis Austin, these granulocyte inclusions are without a doubt the largest and the coarsest. Together with the exceptionally rare storage in the lymphocytes, these alterations are virtually unmistakable.

In contrast, the *bone marrow* findings are unconspicuous and diagnostically much less helpful, at least as far as can yet be determined. In our own investigations, they were generally restricted to fine granular inclusions in the reticulum cells (Fig. 20) and osteoblasts. Reliable reports are not often found in the literature [10, 43], but the few that exist appear to agree with our findings.

The so-called Dale variant [6, 56] which we were able to examine in five patients, cannot be distinguished hematomorphologically from classic MPSosis IV.

19a 19b

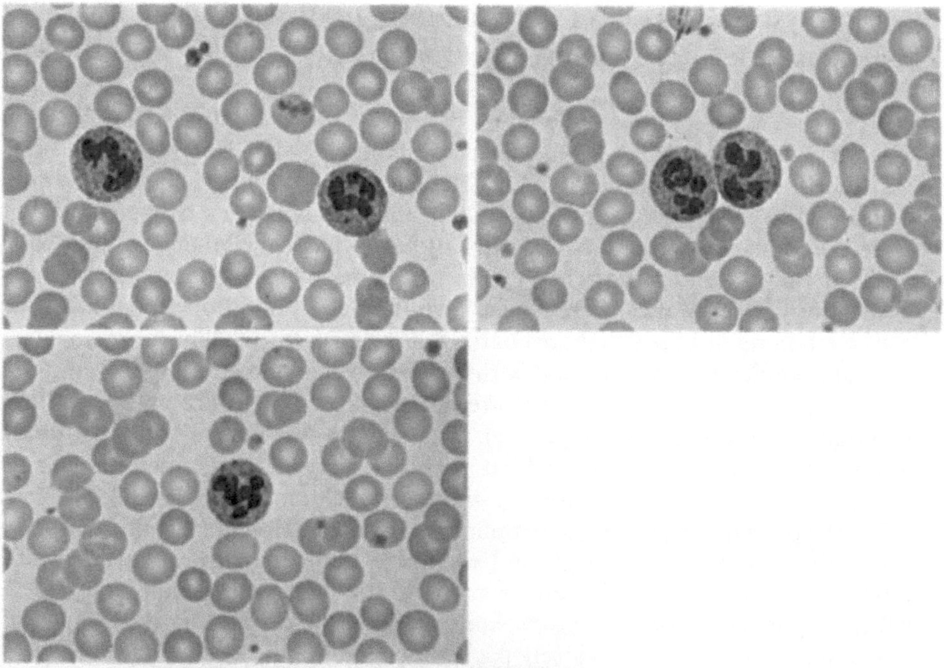

19c

20

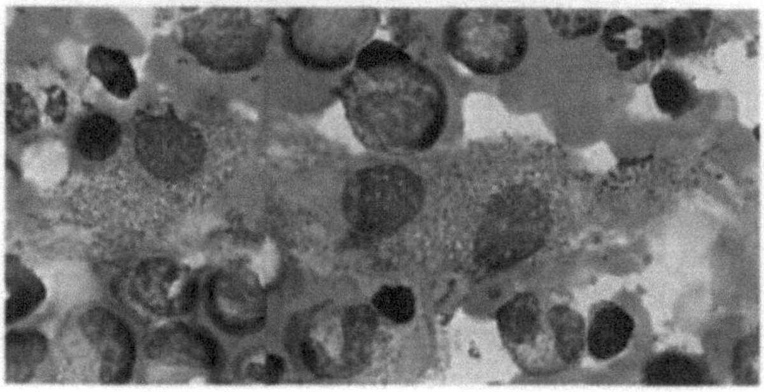

**Fig. 19a–c.** MPSosis IV. Blood. Sparse, coarse, very pronounced inclusions in neutrophilic polymorphs.

**Fig. 20.** MPSosis IV. Reticulum cells in bone marrow. Fine granular, only moderately dense storage.

## **Mucopolysaccharidosis VI** (Arylsulfatase B Deficiency) Synonym: Maroteaux-Lamy Syndrome [32]

The changes in the *blood leukocytes* correspond to what is commonly known as Alder's granulation anomaly (Fig. 21). The excessively dense and sometimes coarse granulation always present in all neutrophils is very conspicuous, but the eosinophils are even more markedly altered (Alder called them "pseudobasophils"). For the most part they exhibit a coarse to very coarse, occasionally even lumpy, dense, always red-violet granulation. In addition, there are some cells containing granules that are coarse but greenish tinged. There are no eosinophilic granules that are normal with respect to size and staining. In contrast, the basophils exhibit granules that are never coarsened but are greatly reduced in number and/or size (Fig. 21d, e). The monocytes behave similarly to the granulocytes; as a rule they exhibit dense to very dense, sometimes coarse, and occasionally even polymorphic inclusions. Compared with the MPSoses I–III, the percentage of storage lymphocytes is lower. However, somewhat more often, the granules are coarse, and the large number of granules per cell is especially prominent. Incidentally, it is worth noting that the small lymphocyte, which is almost devoid of cytoplasm, is frequently affected as well, in which case numerous granules lie closely packed around the nucleus (Fig. 21g).

Besides the granulocytes (Fig. 22) and monocytes in the blood smear already described, the other storage phenomena which occur in the *bone marrow* are comparatively poor. The reticulum cells are only partially affected and, as far as can be judged, altered to a lesser degree than in MPSosis I–H and II. In the plasma cells, only fine and more or less sparse granules can be demonstrated.

The findings derived from two adult sisters with a clinically and radiologically mild variant of type VI have proved difficult to interpret. The very dense granulation of the neutrophils and monocytes is found here also. But the otherwise characteristic red-violet granules in the eosinophils, all of which show storage, are missing, and the granules are greenish. The diminished granulation in the basophils appears less distinct.

**Fig. 21a–g.** MPSosis VI. Blood.

- **a** Neutrophilic polymorphs with very dense but relatively fine granulation.
- **b** Eosinophil with clearly coarsened granules of different colors.
- **c** Eosinophil with very coarse, red-violet granulation.
- **d, e** Basophils. The number, size, and intensity of staining of granules are clearly diminished.
- **f** Monocyte with numerous, reddish granules; the granulation is, however, not as dense as in the neutrophilic granulocytes.
- **g** Lymphocyte with little cytoplasm and numerous granules of different sizes.

**Fig. 22a, b.** MPSosis VI. Neutrophilic and eosinophilic granulocytes in bone marrow. Most impressive is the black-violet storage in the immature eosinophils.

21a 21b 21c

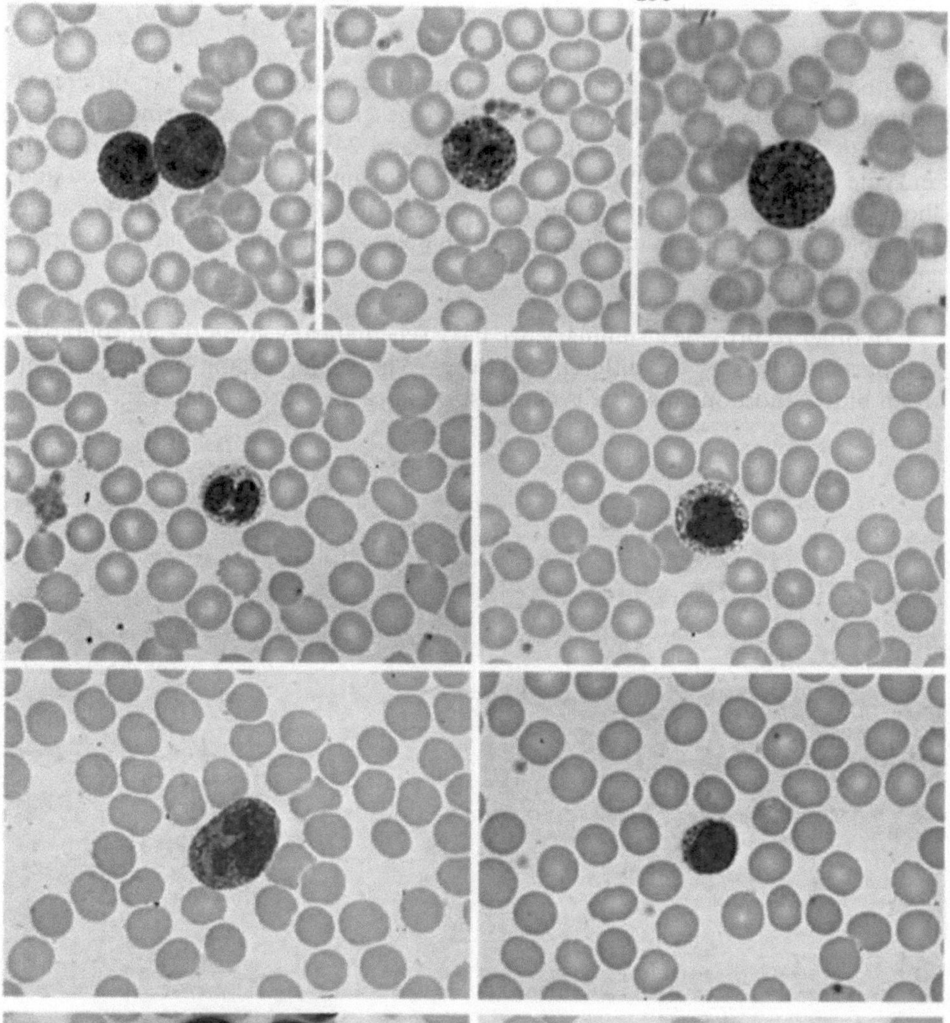

21d 21e

21f 21g

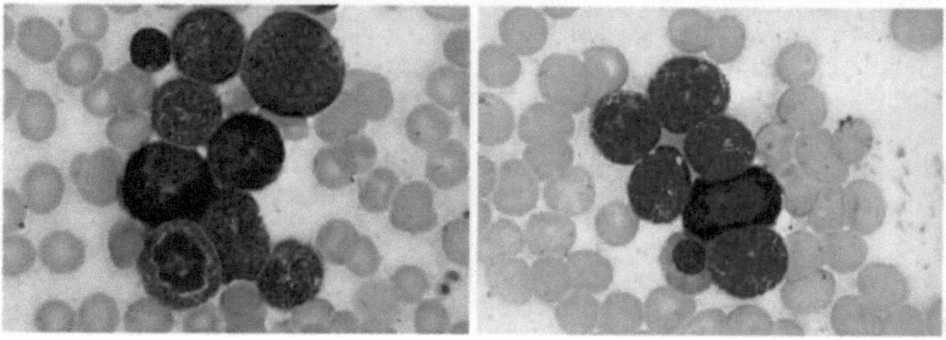

22a 22b

## **Mucopolysaccharidosis VII** (β-Glucuronidase Deficiency) [55]

On the basis of preparations taken from three patients, no clear difference between the blood and bone marrow changes in MPSosis VI and those in MPSosis VII could be determined (Figs. 23 and 24), despite the very different enzyme defects involved. We also had the opportunity of examining blood and bone marrow preparations taken from case I of GIBAUD et al. [16]. We were not able to ascertain any morphological changes and up till now have no explanation for this.

In order to provide a summary, we have schematically given the morphological particularities of the different MPSoses. The distinguishing marker cell for both blood and bone marrow is emphasized in each disorder (Fig. 25a, b).

23a 23b

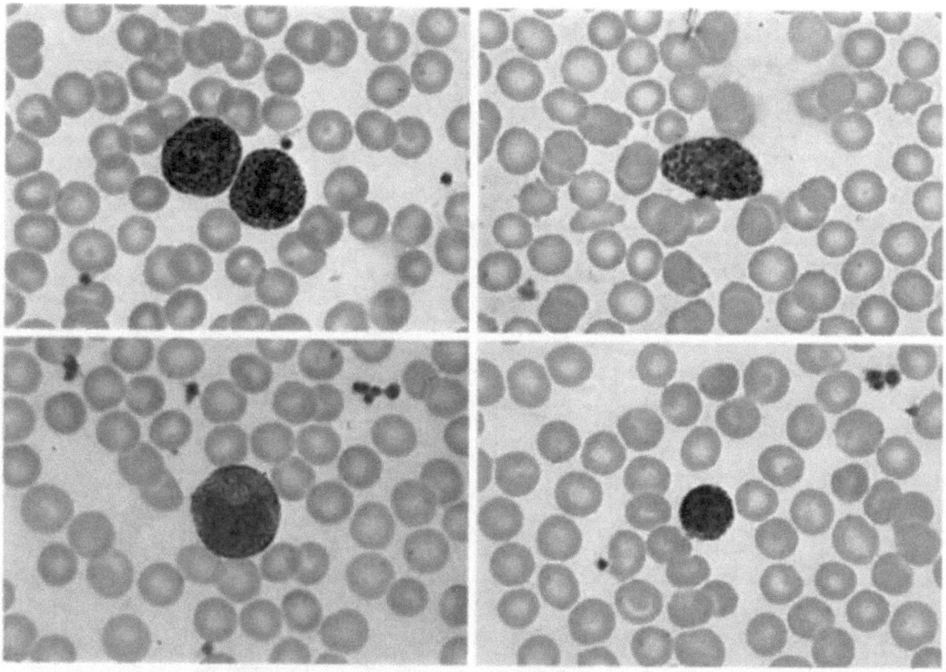

23c 23d

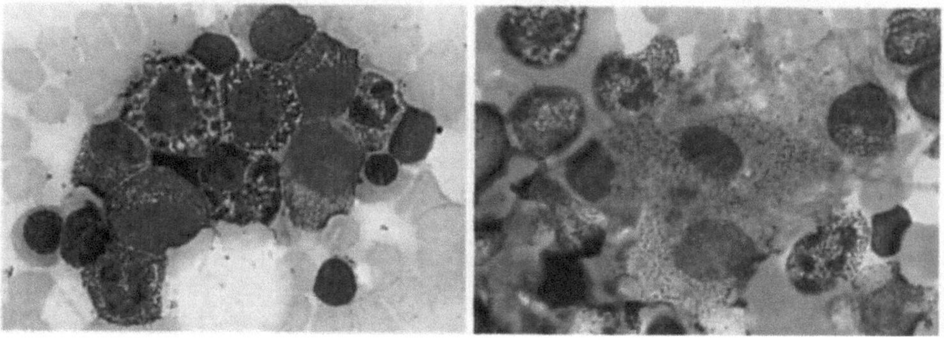

24a 24b

**Fig. 23a–d.** MPSosis VII. Blood.
**a** Neutrophilic polymorphs with very dense, but relatively fine granulation.
**b** Eosinophil with coarse red-violet granulation.
**c** Dense, fine granulation in monocyte.
**d** Lymphocyte with little cytoplasm and numerous fine granules crowded round the nucleus.

**Fig. 24a, b.** MPSosis VII. Bone marrow.
**a** Eosinophils and neutrophils with typical storage phenomena.
**b** Reticulum cells with only moderately dense, fine granulation.

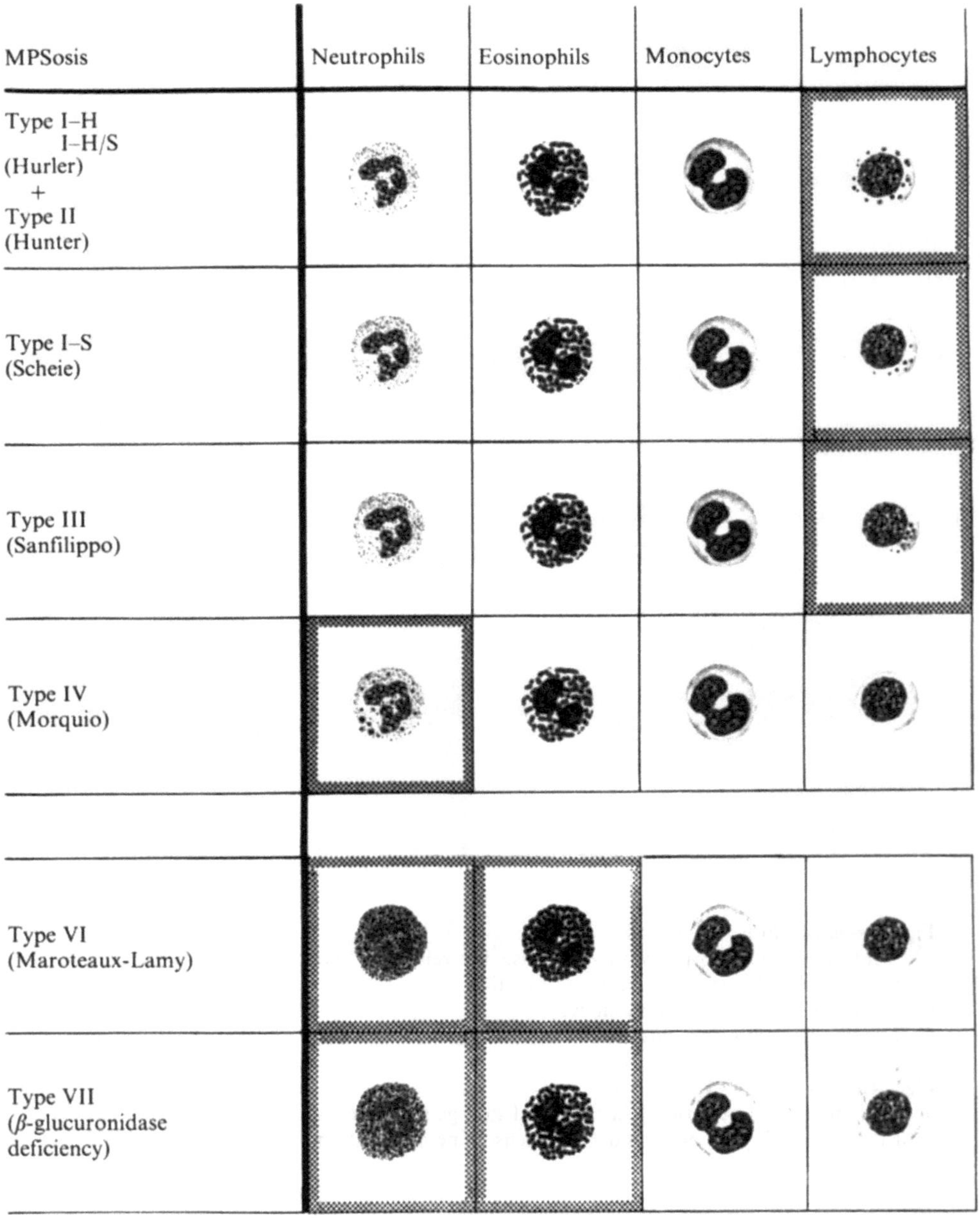


**Fig. 25 a, b.** Schematic survey of morphologically characteristic cells (marker cells) in MPSoses.
**a** Blood. Marker cells bordered.

## BONE MARROW

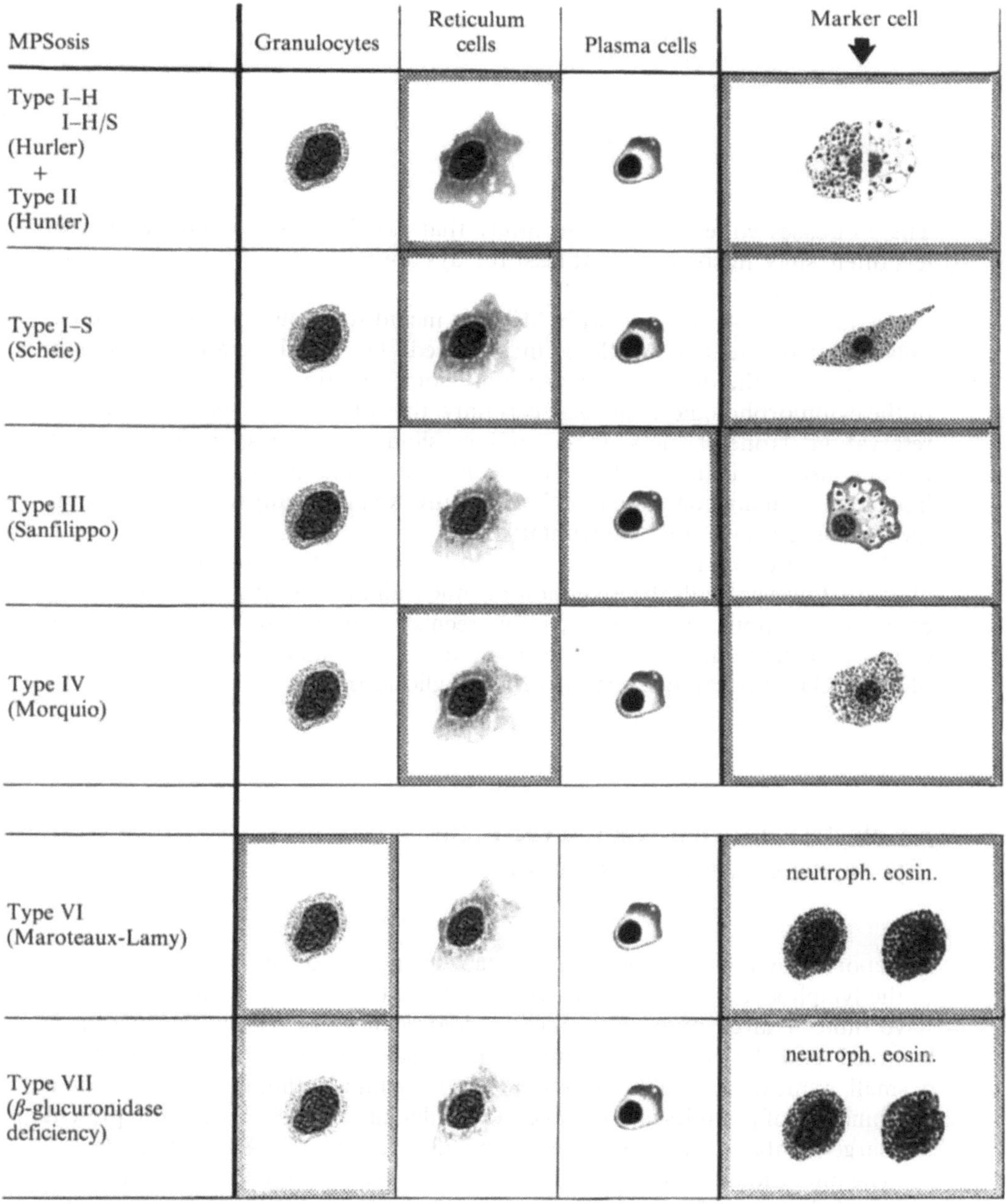


**b** Bone marrow. Cell line derived from and marker cells bordered.

# Mucolipidoses

These diseases either occur more rarely than the MPSoses or are recognized less often, since in some cases at least the dysmorphism is clinically less marked or even absent.

In fact, the 68 patients with MLoses included in our material represent only about one-half of MPSoses investigated. The small number of cases in some forms of the diseases may well raise some question as to the significance of the cytomorphological changes; certainly, the valuation should be made with reservation. None the less, these findings should be discussed, first, as they are of considerable importance, and second, since descriptions and illustrations have been virtually nonexistent in the literature, and not many details concerning these disorders have been known until now.

The MLoses are analogous to the MPSoses in that the eosinophils are often altered. However, with the exception of mucosulfatidosis Austin and I-cell disease, there is not only a coarse, gray-greenish granulation but also a partial decrease in the number and size of granules. These changes are diagnostically of no crucial importance except in $G_{M1}$-gangliosidosis I.

## **β-Galactosidase Deficiency, Type I** [26]
(Synonym: $G_{M1}$-Gangliosidosis I)

As reported by most authors, the most conspicuous change in the *blood* occurs in the lymphocytes. A large proportion of them (mean 88%; range 74%–93%) have quite a large number of fine or coarse vacuoles. Often the plasma is enlarged, and the vacuoles accumulate paranuclearly (Fig. 26d). Furthermore, a small number of lymphocytes (1%–2%) contain pathologic granules or a combination of granules and vacuoles. Granules and/or vacuoles are also present in a large number of the monocytes (mean 73%; range 60%–87%) (Fig. 26e–g).

The alterations occurring in the eosinophils have been neglected until now, although they are of special interest (Fig. 26a–c). A small number of granules here are coarse and stained gray-greenish, while the remaining granules are diminished in number, size, and stainability. Thus, by comparison, the former appear more multicolored, although they are in fact more pallid than normal eosinophils. The latter are virtually impossible to find in the blood smear.

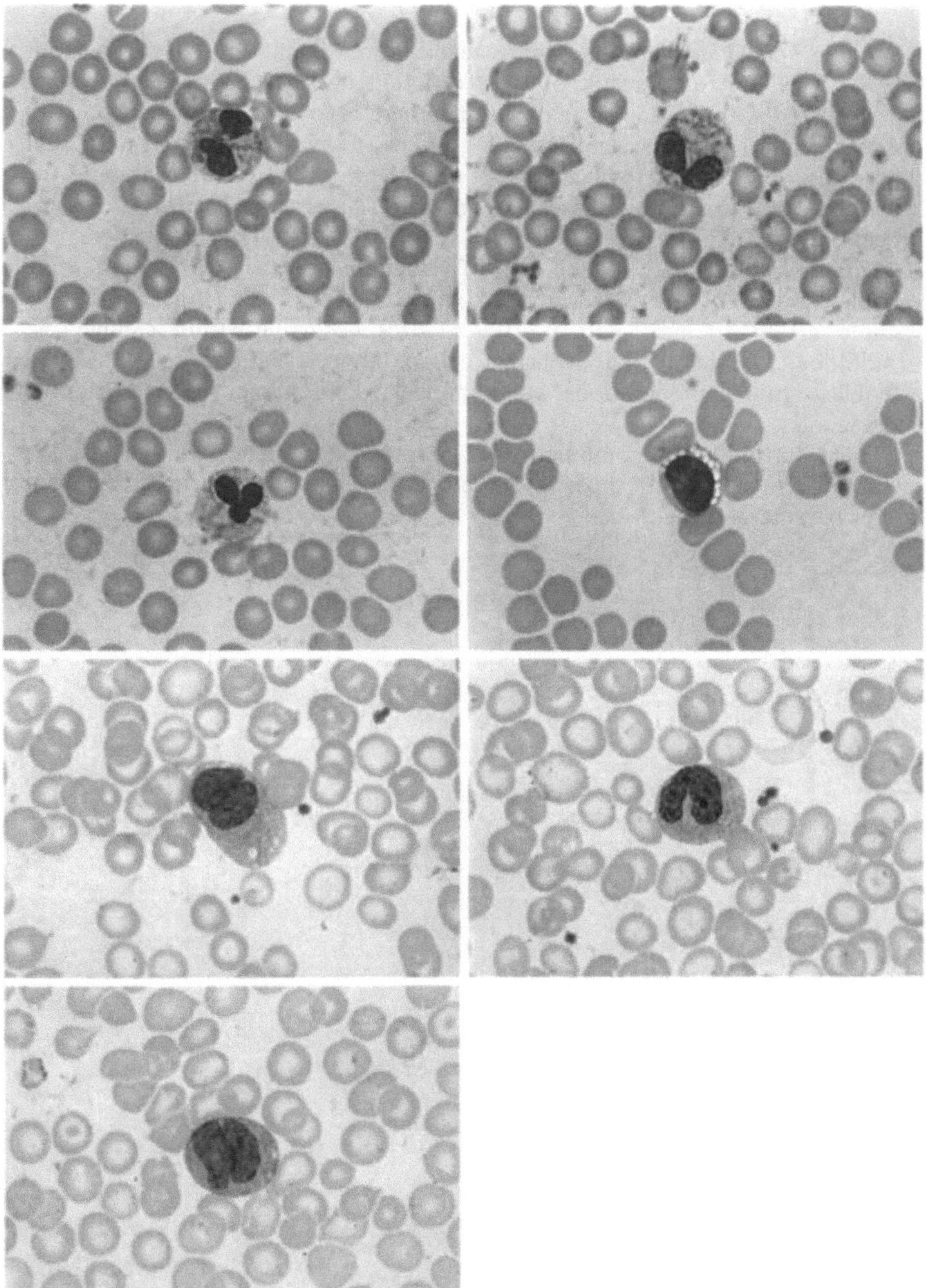

26a 26b 26c 26d 26e 26f 26g

**Fig. 26a–g.** *β*-Galactosidase deficiency I. Blood.

**a–c** Eosinophils which have nearly lost their original characteristic features. The granules are diminished in number, size, and stainability. The granules appear more colorful, but the cells as a whole more pallid than normal.

**d** Lymphocyte with coarse, distinct vacuoles.

**e–g** Monocytes with vacuoles, with fine granules, and with both.

In the *bone marrow,* it is again the eosinophils that are so conspicuous (Fig. 27a, b), but as a result of their different ages (the changes becoming more marked with advancing maturation), there is considerable variation with respect to color, number and size of granules. It was more by chance that these cells were noticed by SERINGE et al. [54] in 1968, but at that time the authors did not realize that these were eosinophils altered as a result of storage processes.

Finally, large, round storage cells of reticulohistiocytary origin containing vacuoles, granules, or both, are found in the bone marrow (Fig. 27c–e). The vacuoles are for the most part of different sizes, occurring within a single cell. In addition, a fraction of the plasma cells is always slightly vacuolated. All osteoblasts in the preparations we examined exhibit numerous fine granules and vacuoles.

To recapitulate, the combination of storage phenomena exhibited by the eosinophils, together with those in the reticulum cells, can be regarded as absolutely characteristic.

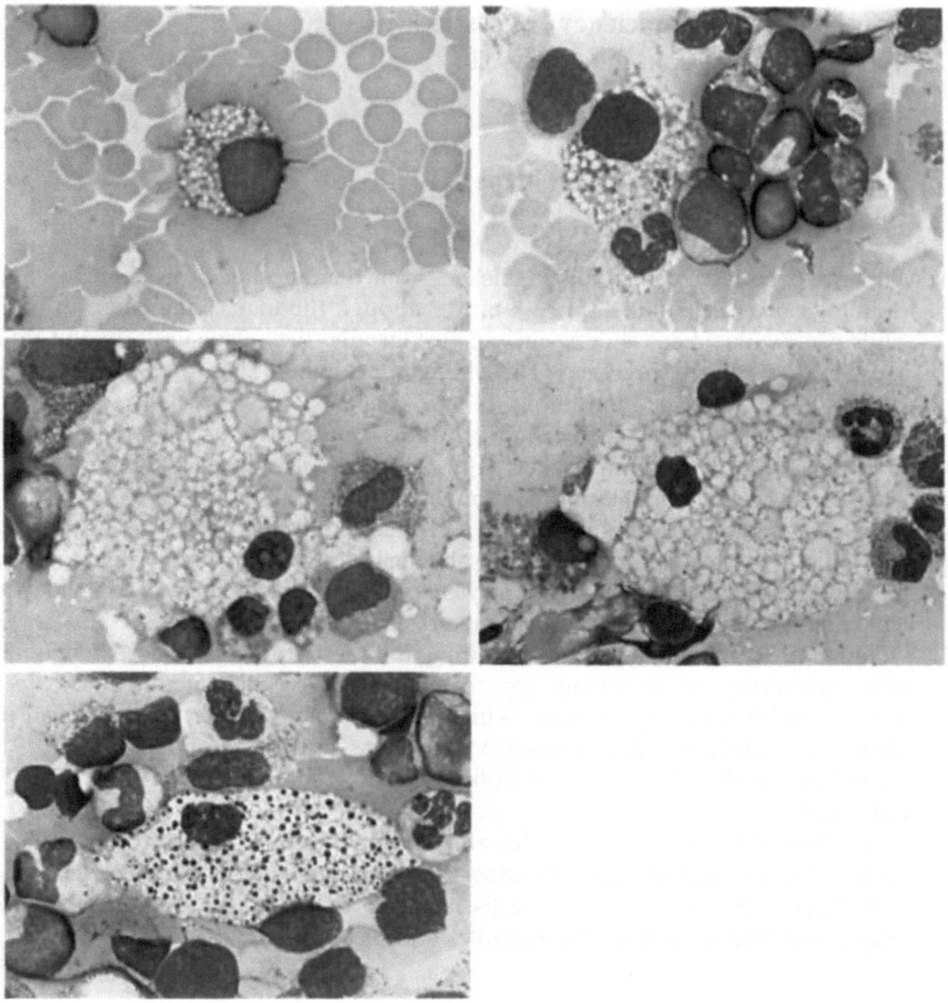

27a 27b 27c 27d 27e

**Fig. 27 a–e.** $\beta$-Galactosidase deficiency I. Bone marrow.

**a–b** Immature eosinophils with pronounced loss of granules.

**c–d** Reticulum cells filled with vacuoles of varying size in between which are single, fine granules.

**e** Reticulum cell with predominantly coarse granular storage.

## $\beta$-Galactosidase Deficiency, Types II [7]
Synonym: $G_{M1}$-Gangliosidosis II

and

## $\beta$-Galactosidase Deficiency, Type III [30, 38]

These two diseases can be distinguished from one another both clinically and radiologically (see Table 2, pp. 8–9), even though the underlying cause in both cases is a $\beta$-galactosidase deficiency. Cytologically, they also similarly and thus can here be treated together. The changes brought about by these diseases have not been described until now.

In the *blood smear*, a fine, more or less dense vacuolation predominates in about 50% of the lymphocytes (Fig. 28). Granular deposits seldom occur. There are also fine vacuoles in the monocytes (40%–60%).

The characteristic marker cell is to be found in the *bone marrow* (Fig. 29a–e). It is unique in this class and does not occur in any other storage disease. (We have seen similar cells only in a 4-year-old patient with chronic myelocytic leukemia.) This marker cell is characterized by the peculiar light blue – we would like to call it sky blue – staining of the cytoplasm. These reticulum cells, measuring up to 40 µm, are covered with very delicate, netlike, wide-meshed, reddish structures, upon which fine, reddish granules are arranged in chains. The acid phosphatase and PAS reactions are strongly positive (Fig. 29f, g), indicating the presence of glycolipids of low solubility and is, of course, not specific.

Compared to these marker cells, all other findings are of minor importance: there are also reticulum cells with either sparse or dense and usually fine granulation. Vacuolation of the plasma cells is rather rare. On the other hand, most osteoblasts contain sparse, fine vacuoles and/or granules.

**Fig. 28a, b.** $\beta$-Galactosidase deficiency II. Blood lymphocytes with relatively sparse, fine vacuoles.

**Fig. 29a–g.** $\beta$-Galactosidase deficiency II. Reticulum cells in bone marrow.

**a–e** Light to medium blue cells, which we describe as sky blue, covered with very delicate, netlike, wide-meshed, reddish structures upon which very fine granules are arranged.

**f** Very strongly positive acid phosphatase reaction (even though the preparation was 1 year old upon reaction).

**g** PAS reaction strongly positive.

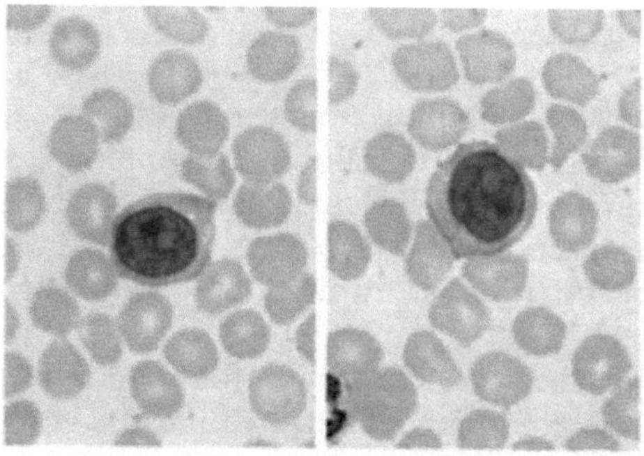

28a, b

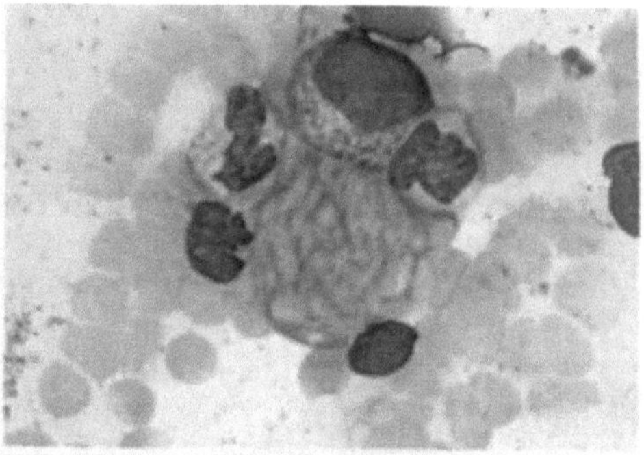

29a

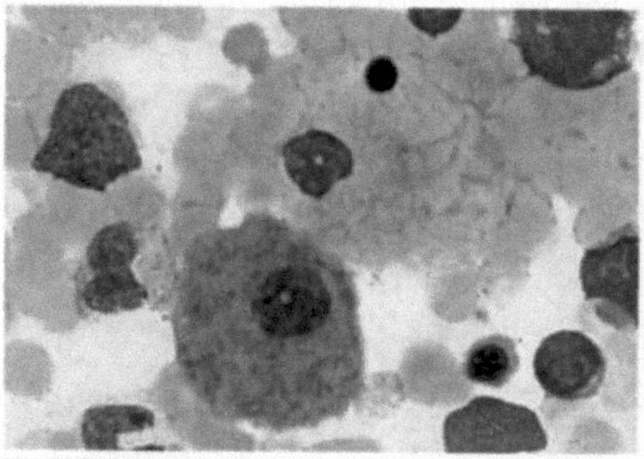

29b

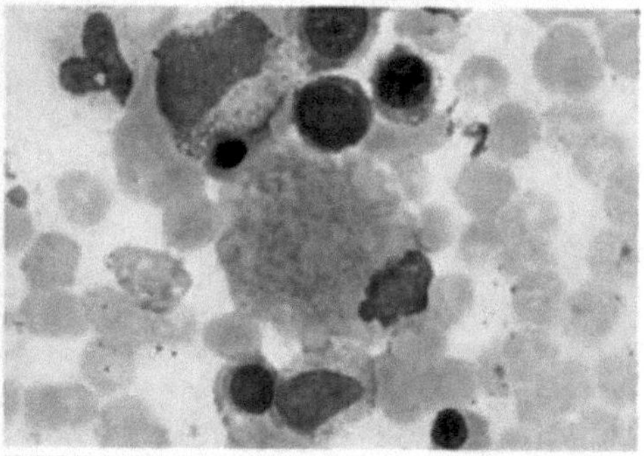

29c

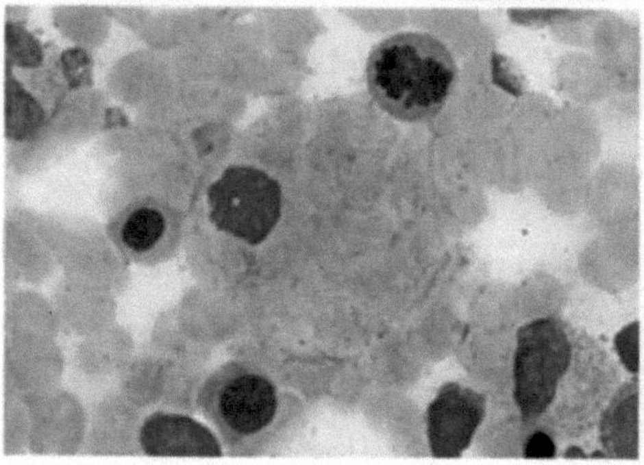

29d

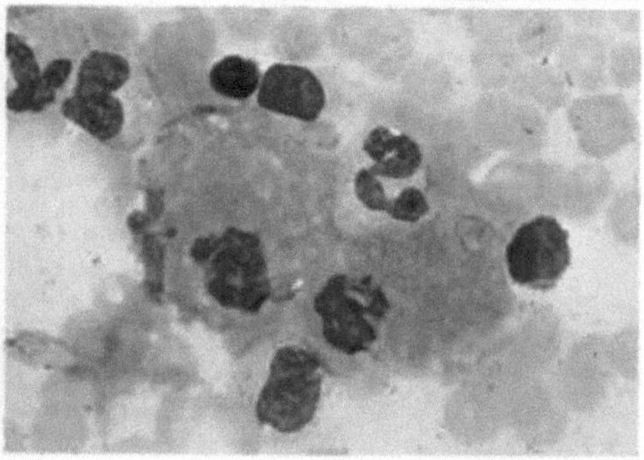

29e

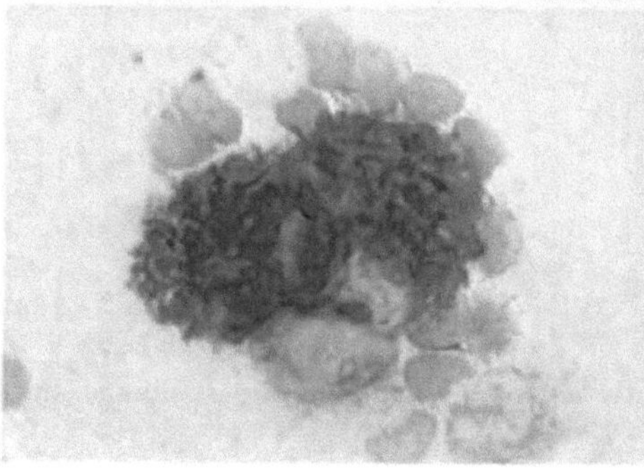

29f

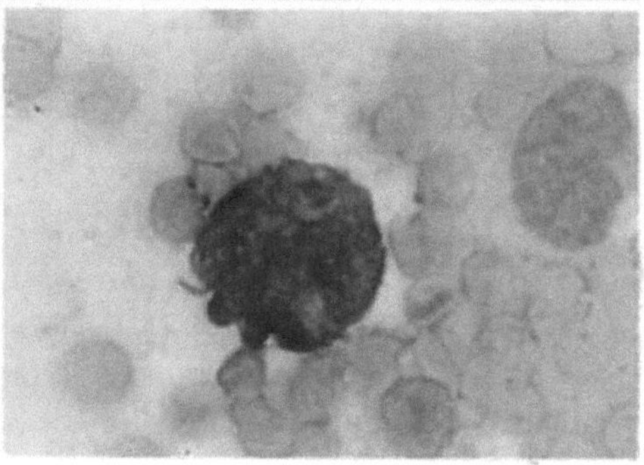

29g

## **Fucosidosis** (α-L-Fucosidase Deficiency) [9]

Preparations from only one patient were available for examination.

In *blood smears* taken a year apart, we found 11% and 30% lymphocytes respectively with fine vacuolation. Compared to β-galactosidase deficiency I, for example, or even mannosidosis, the vacuoles are as a rule sparser, more indistinct, and more often irregularly distributed throughout the plasma (Fig. 30).

About 50% of the reticulum cells of the *marow* exhibit "foam cell"-like changes (Fig. 31 a–c); i.e., vacuoles are the predominant feature, and the granules are, if present, fine and sparse. Another, smaller proportion of the reticulum cells show only granular storage with wide variation in intensity (Fig. 31 d, e). Changes in the plasma cells are negligible. Osteoblasts were missing in the preparations.

**Fig. 30 a–c.** Fucosidosis. Blood lymphocytes with fine, usually sparse, and partially indistinct vacuoles.

**Fig. 31 a–e.** Fucosidosis. Reticulum cells in bone marrow.
**a, b** Predominantly coarse, in part also fine vacuolated, distended cells.
**c** Mixed, fine vacuolated, and fine granular storage.
**d, e** Exclusively granular inclusions which are particularly fine in **d**.

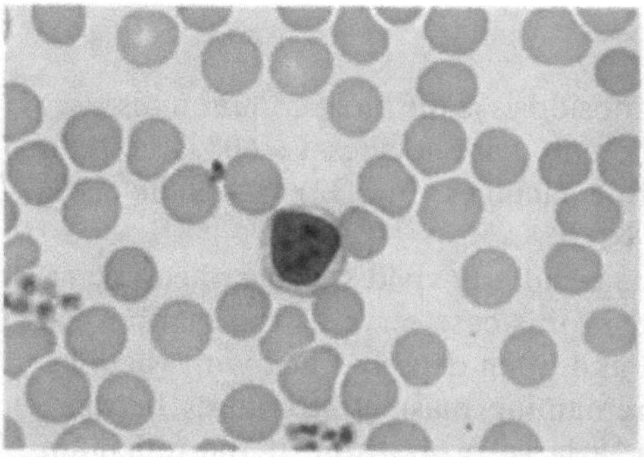

30a

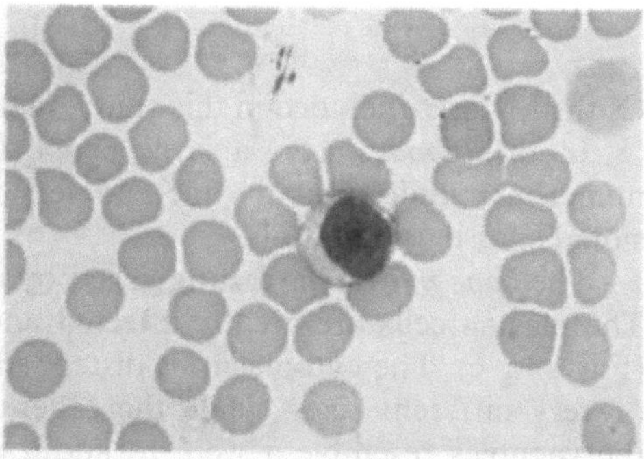

30b

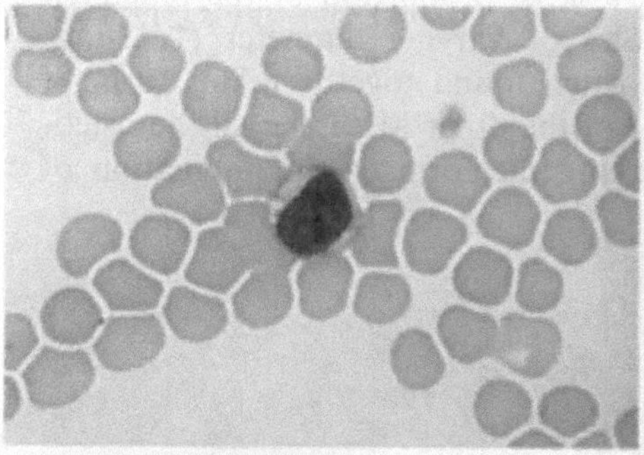

30c

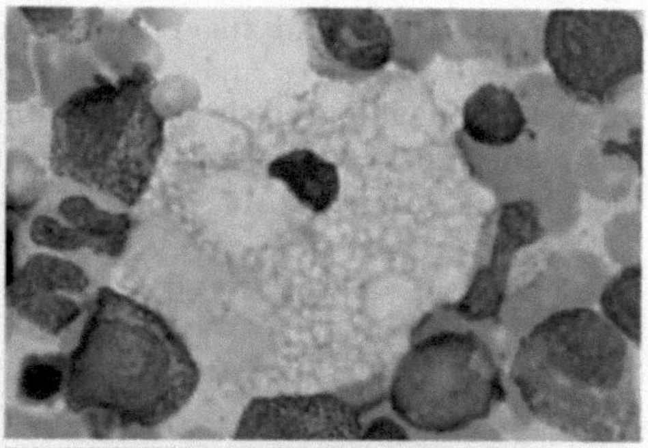

31a

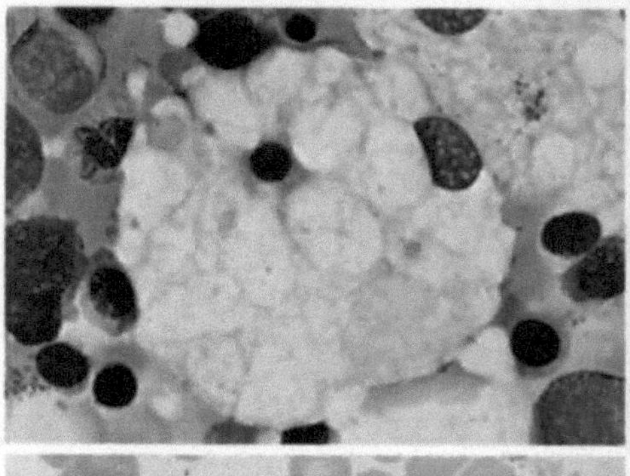

31b

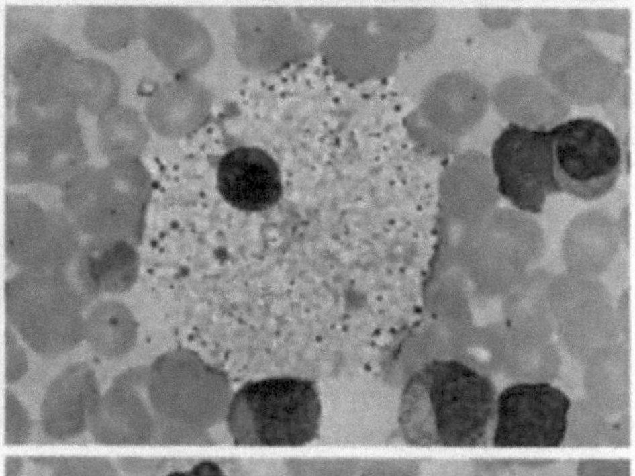

31c

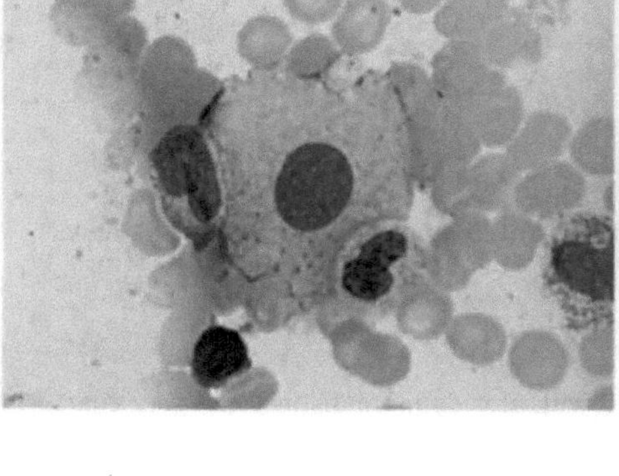

31d

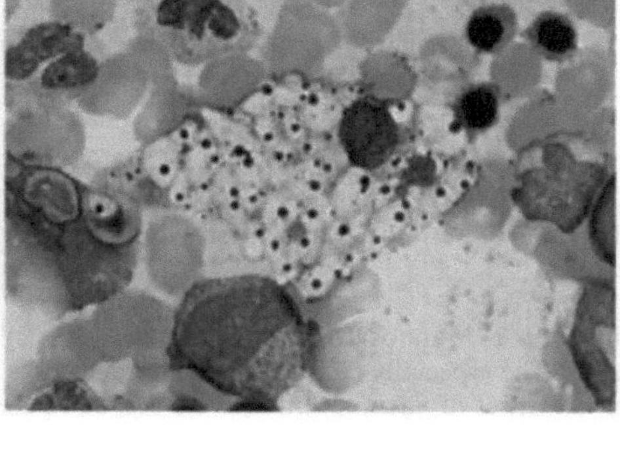

31e

## **Mannosidosis** ($\beta$-D-Mannosidase Deficiency ) [39]

Of the MLoses included in this study, mannosidosis is the most common disease.

In the *blood smear*, a large proportion of lymphocytes (~60%) contain numerous, predominantly fine and very fine vacuoles (Fig. 32) as well as occasional sparse granulation.

The *bone marrow* is distinguished by its peculiarly vivid storage phenomena. The plasma cells are greatly affected and in this case serve as the marker cell (Fig. 33a–c). The cytoplasm is distended and often densely filled with vacuoles of very different sizes, while the other remaining plasmic structures between the vacuoles resemble a web. In additon, a large proportion of the reticulum cells are enlarged and filled with vacuoles of varying diameter (1–11 μm) (Fig. 33d, e). Vacuoles and granules are often found together. This form of storage in reticulum cells is similar to that of the other MLoses. All the osteoblasts are altered, the changes usually taking the form of a combination of vacuoles and granules.

**Fig. 32a–c.** Mannosidosis. Blood lymphocytes with relatively numerous, more or less fine vacuoles.

**Fig. 33a–e.** Mannosidosis. Bone marrow.

**a–c** The especially characteristic plasma cells.

**a** Onset of vacuolation at *lower left* compared with already more distinct and very coarse vacuoles, *above right*.

**b, c** Very numerous, distinct, uniform vacuoles, widened cytoplasm.

**d, e** Reticulum cells with mixed, fine to very coarse vacuolation. Additionally, in **e**, pale blue plaques and cell phagocytosis.

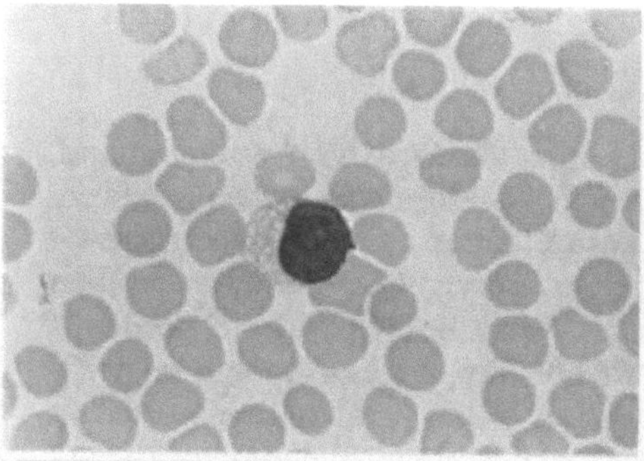
32a

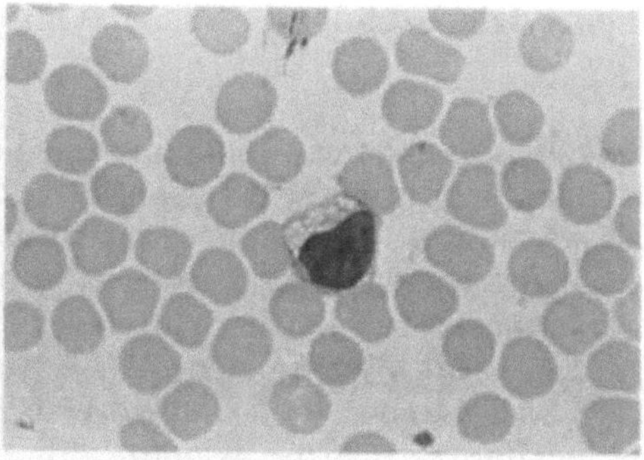
32b

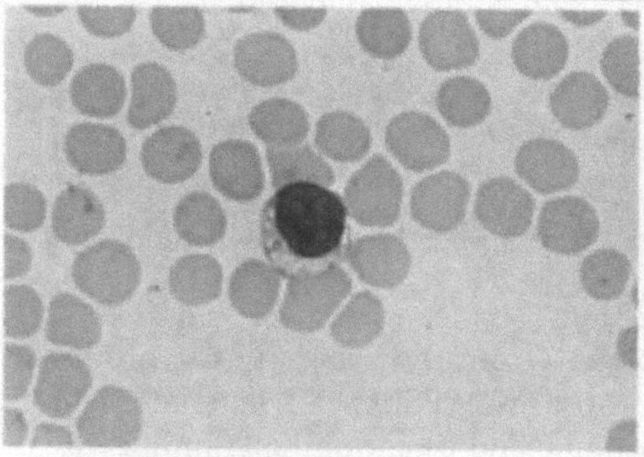
32c

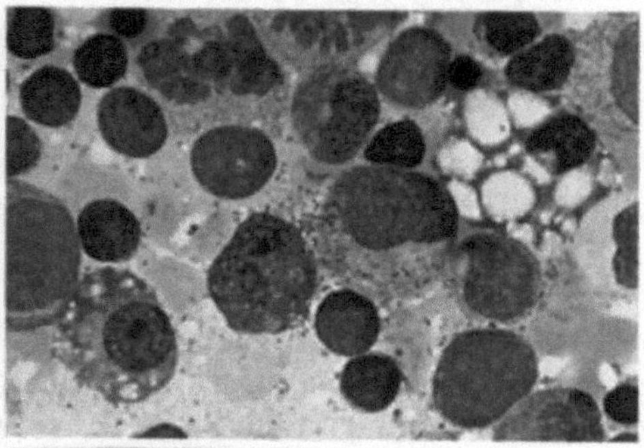
33a

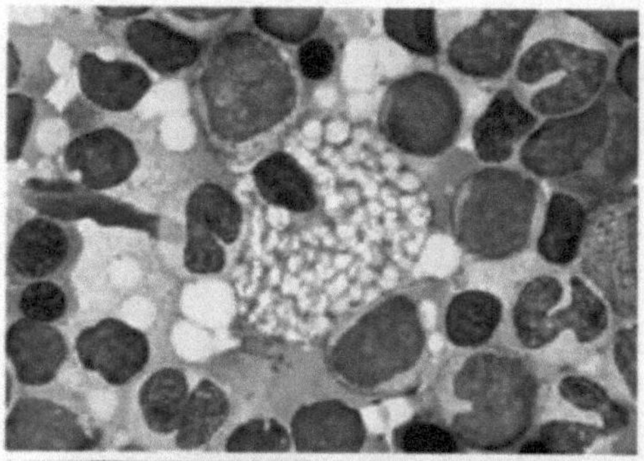
33b

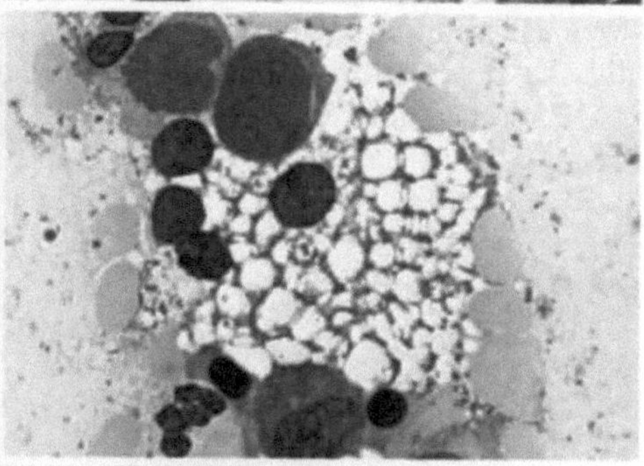
33c

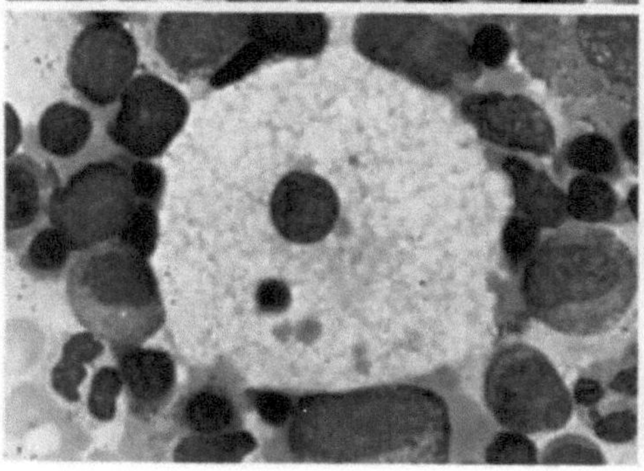
33d

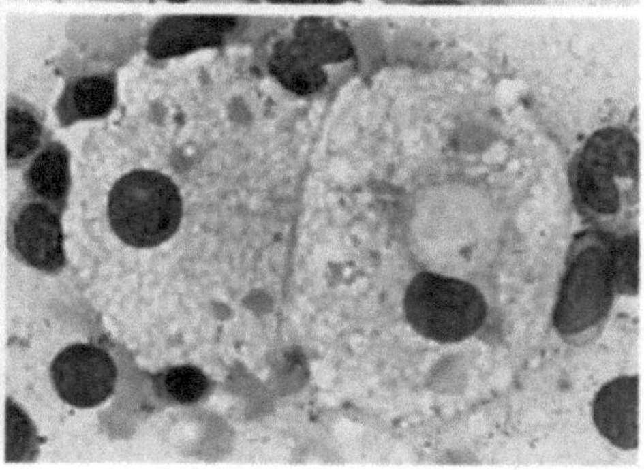
33e

## **Aspartylglucosaminuria** (Aspartylglucosaminidase Deficiency) [42]

This disease is apparently not only rare, but hardly known at all outside Finland, and then only in isolated cases [5, 15, 23, 42]. In the *blood smears,* we were able to confirm the data given in the literature concerning the occurrence of vacuolated lymphocytes. The vacuoles are not very numerous and are fine, or even very fine, and in part indistinct. Often, the cytoplasmic border is broadened (Fig. 34). Unfortunately, we did not have access to bone marrow preparations, and to our knowledge such findings have not been reported in the literature. It can be assumed, however, that storage phenomena of any kind may likewise be demonstrated.

## **Mucosulfatidosis Austin** (Arylsulfatase A and B Deficiency) [2]

Morphologically, this disease differs completely from the others in the group. The *blood smear* findings are identical to those in MPSosis VI and VII, i.e., pronounced, dense granulation in all neutrophilic and eosinophilic granulocytes as well as in almost all monocytes and in about half of the lymphocytes (Fig. 35). Only the proportion of basophils with diminished granulation is lower than for MPSosis VI and VII.

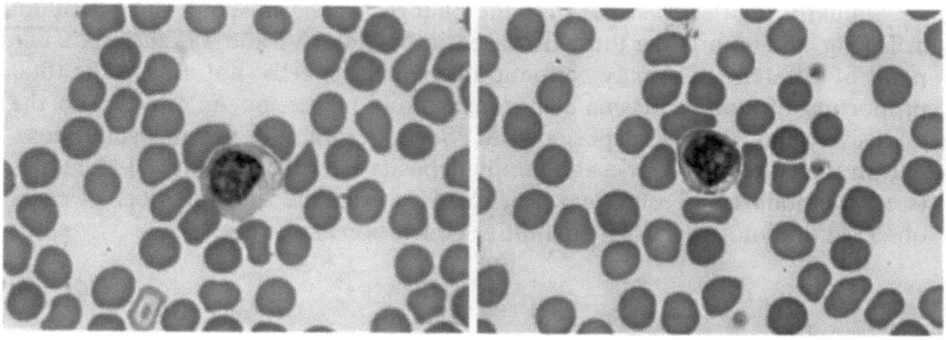

34a 34b

**Fig. 34a, b.** Aspartylglucosaminuria. Blood lymphocytes with fine, relatively sparse vacuoles; in **a** arranged like grapes (Wright staining).

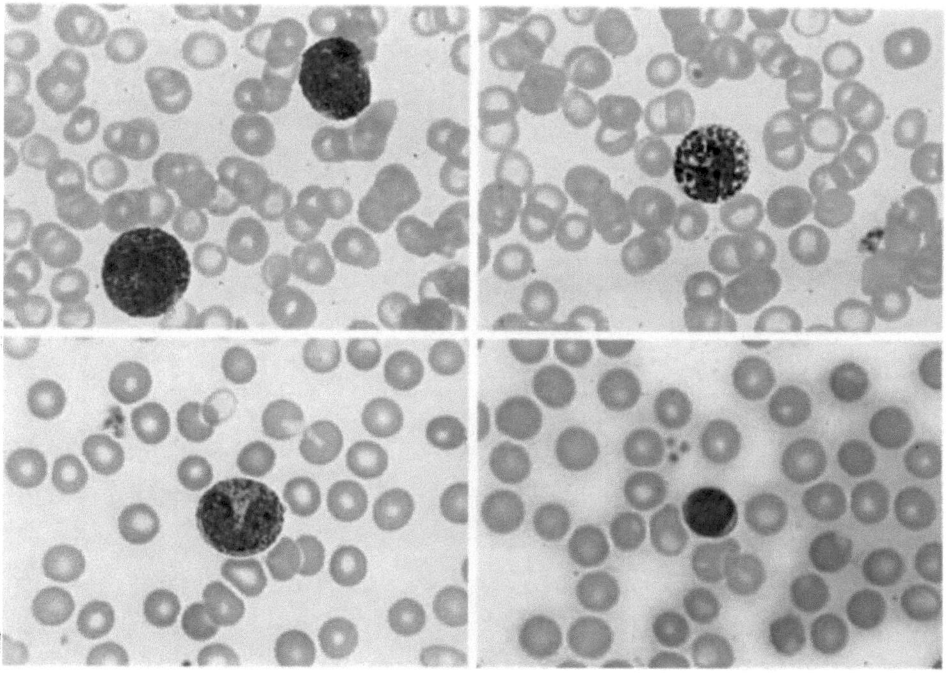

35a 35b 35c 35d

**Fig. 35a–d.** Mucosulfatidosis. Blood.

**a** Heavy, dense granulation in neutrophilic polymorphs.
**b** Eosinophil with very coarse, red-violet granulation.
**c** Less numerous, relatively fine granules in monocytes.
**d** Small lymphocyte with moderately dense, very fine granulation.

Similarly, in the *bone marrow,* the changes in the myeloid and reticulum cells (Fig. 36a–c) are like those observed in MPSosis VI and VII. One possible point of differentiation may be found in the plasma cells: not only is the total proportion of storing plasma cells considerably higher, but in addition to the exclusively fine grained deposits in MPSosis VI and VII in mucosulfatidosis Austin there are also coarse and lumpy deposits as well as Buhot cell-like types (see "Methods and Techniques", p. 16). However, the small number of cases observed does not permit any definitive conclusions to be drawn.

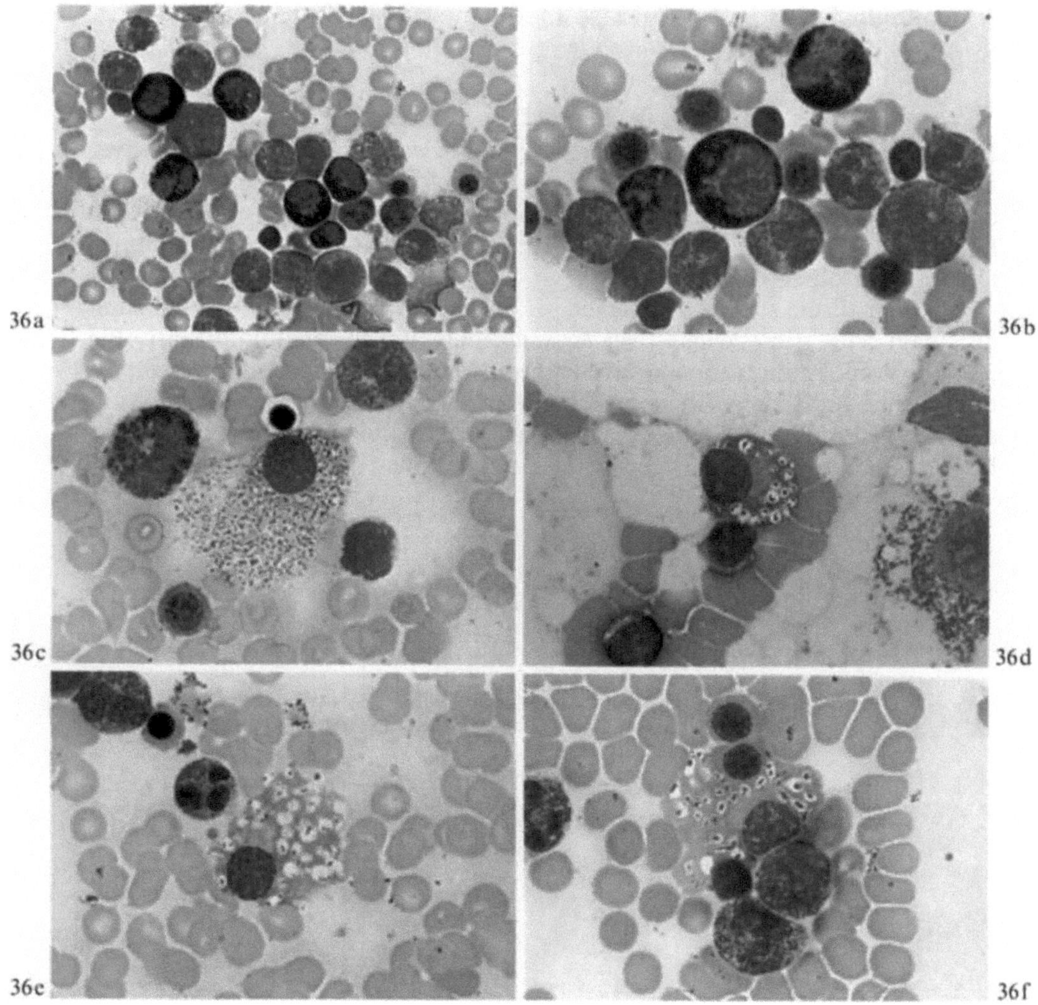


**Fig. 36a–f.** Mucosulfatidosis. Bone marrow.

**a–b** Neutrophilic and eosinophilic granulocytes; particularly impressive is the black-violet storage in the immature eosinophils; (**a** magnification, × 500).

**c** Reticulum cell with relatively dense, fine granulation.

**d–f** Pronounced, polymorphic storage phenomena in plasma cells.

## **Mucolipidosis I** (Neuraminidase Deficiency) [58, 57]
Synonym: Sialidosis

In the *blood smear,* the changes in the lymphocytes (Fig. 37) are qualitatively indistinguishable from those occurring in $\beta$-galactosidase deficiency or mannosidosis. However, quantitatively, the proportion of vacuolated forms is clearly lower (20%–30%). This is also true for monocytes. Granular inclusions are almost never observed.

Peculiar to the storage phenomena in the *bone marrow* is the predominance of "foam cells" (in French, "*cellules spumeuses*") of unusual uniformity (Fig. 38). The vacuolation is comparatively fine and monomorphic, and the juxtaposition of fine and coarse vacuoles is very rare. If present, granular structures are only very discrete. Changes in the plasma cells are insignificant. All osteoblasts contain a mixture of fine vacuoles and granules.

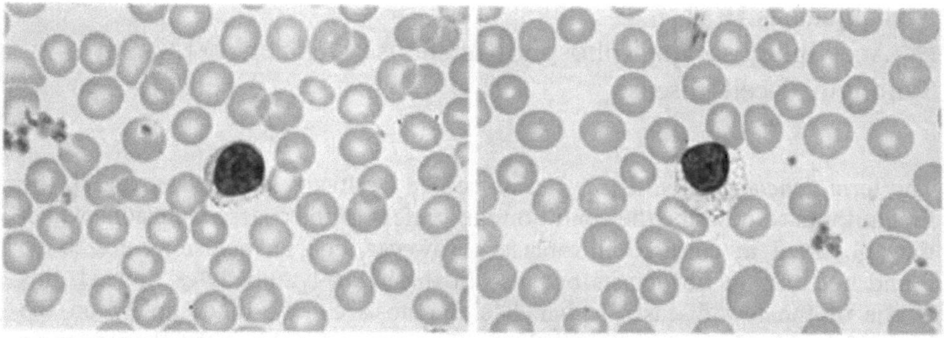

37a 37b

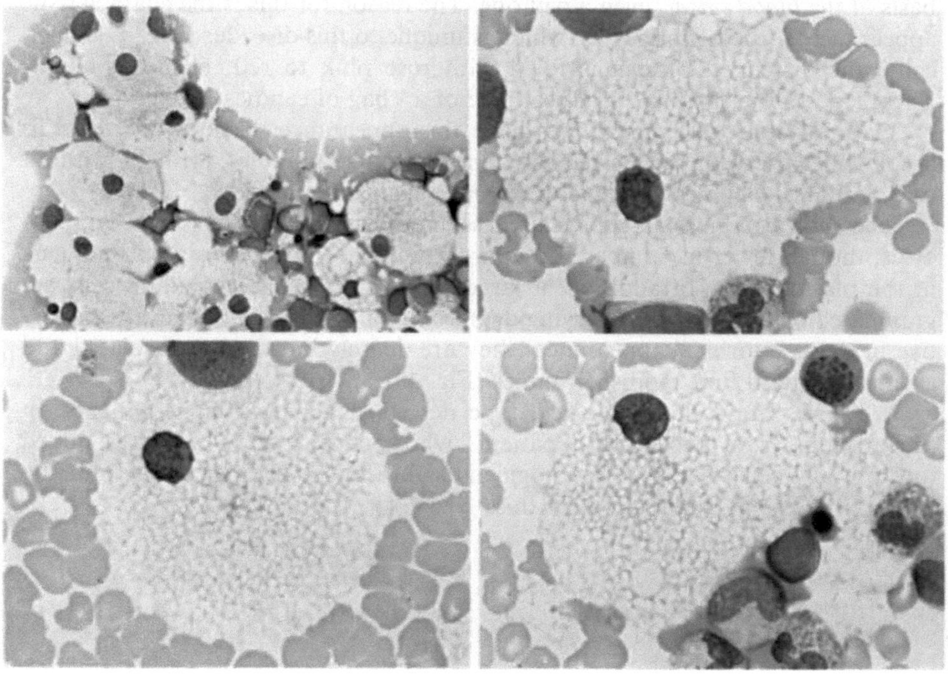

38a 38b 38c 38d

**Fig. 37a, b.** Mucolipidosis I. Blood lymphocytes with varying degrees of relatively fine vacuolation.

**Fig. 38a–d.** Mucolipidosis I. Bone marrow.
**a** Cluster of unusual uniform storage cells (magnification, × 320).
**b–d** Typical "foam cells", i.e., reticulum cells with fine vacuolates of uniform size.

## Mucolipidosis II

(*N*-Acetylglucosaminyl-phosphotransferase Deficiency) [27, 28]
Synonym: I-cell Disease

The term "*inclusion cell disease*" was coined by LEROY and DEMARS [27], the first authors to describe the condition, and refers to the coarse inclusions which they observed in cultured fibroblasts. However, coarse inclusions are to be found not only in fibroblasts but also in the blood lymphocytes. Indeed, this is one of the few diseases in which a diagnosis can be made solely on the basis of the *blood smear,* even a bad one. The reason for this is the characteristic appearance of the lymphocytes, which is unique to this disorder (Fig. 39). Typically, the distended plasma is filled with rose pink to red, roundish lumps. These lend to the plasma the appearance of a "bag of candies" [20].

Naturally, not all lymphocytes have this appearance. Besides this, there is a colorful variety of red or reddish, fine or coarse granules, with or without fine or coarse vacuoles. This picture is once again characteristic.

The *bone marrow* is diagnostically less important. It exhibits similar lymphocytes, though fewer in number and apart from this, similar storage phenomena in the plasma cells. In addition, a large proportion of the reticulum cells are granulated or vacuolated to varying degrees. Finally, the osteoblasts are distinctive in their "morbid" appearance; they are densely but finely vacuolated and as a rule contain fine, reddish granules (Fig. 40).

We have found the cytological type described above in eight patients. In preparations from another five patients whose clinical pictures corresponded to those of I-cell disease, all cytologically significant phenomena were missing. As yet, there is no explanation for this.

**Fig. 39a–e.** Mucolipidosis II. Blood. Peculiarly characteristic aspect of lymphocytes: in the usually enlarged plasma, there are not only fine to moderately coarse, reddish granules but also rose pink to reddish, lump-like inclusions of blurred contour as well as vacuoles. The various mixtures provide a colorful picture ("bag of candies").

**Fig. 40a, b.** Mucolipidosis II. Bone marrow. Particularly marked changes in osteoblasts in form of numerous vacuoles and fine reddish granules.

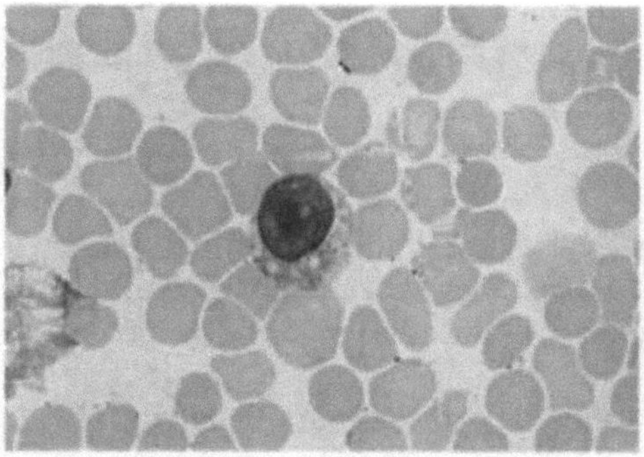
39a

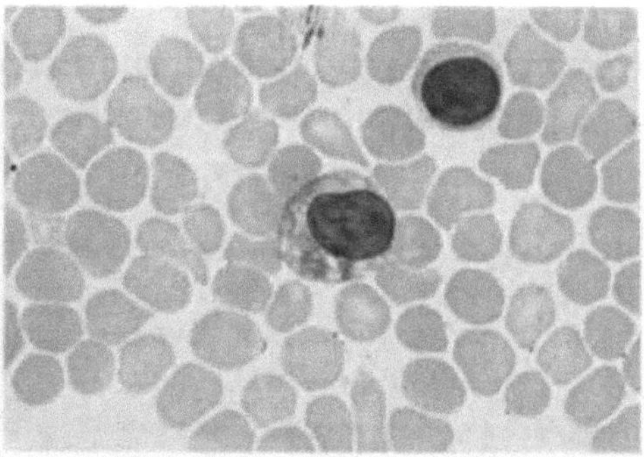
39b

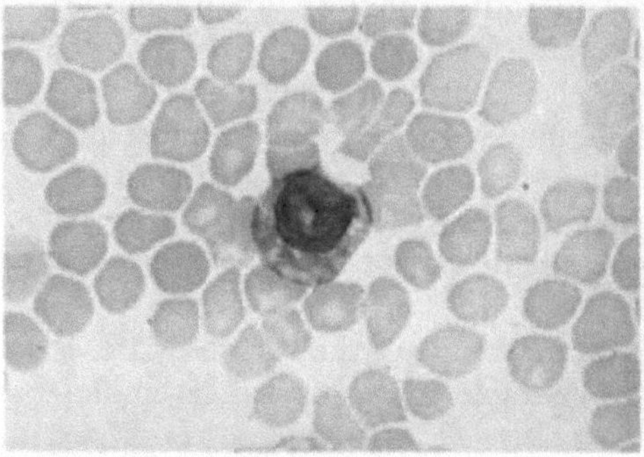
39c

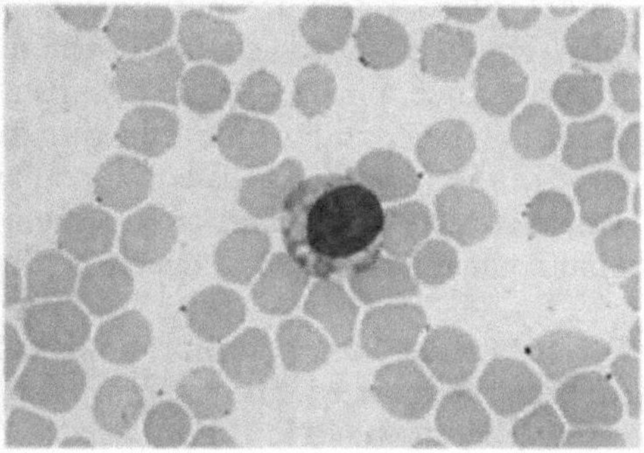
39d

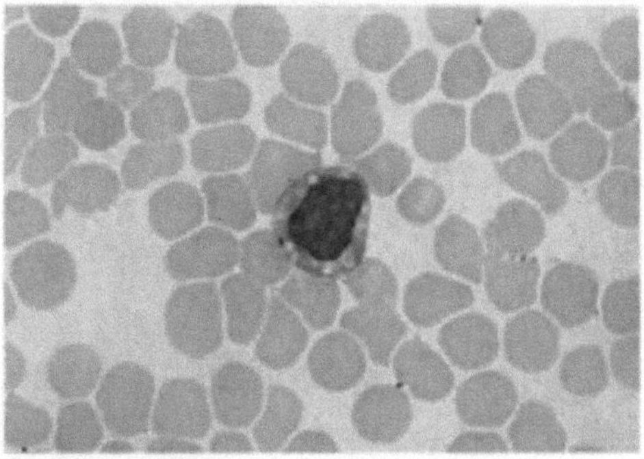
39e

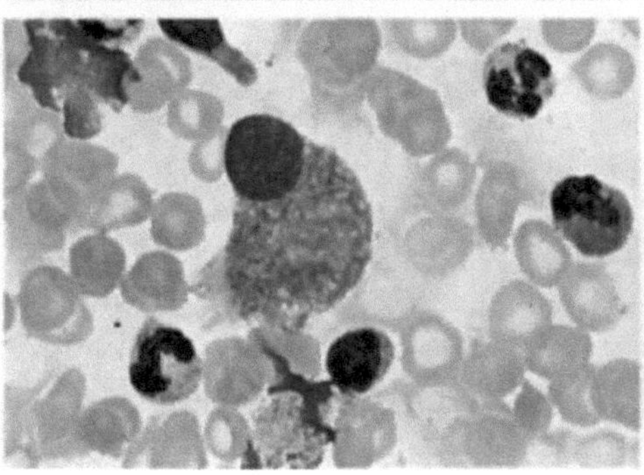
40a

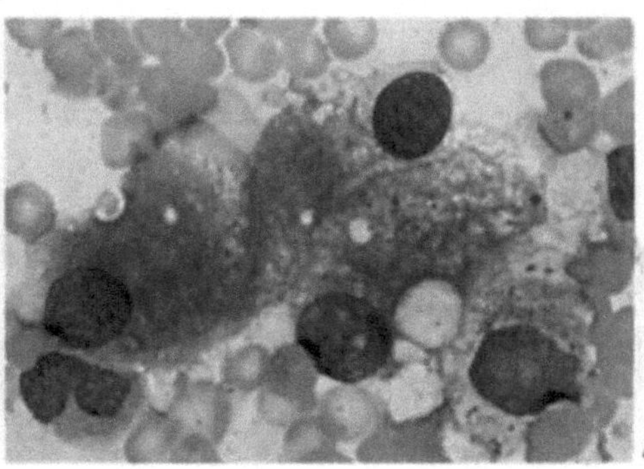
40b

## Mucolipidosis III

(*N*-Acetylglucosaminyl-phosphotransferase Deficiency) [31]
Synonym: Pseudo-polydystrophy

Not only the clinical picture but also the cytological findings of this disease vary. Correspondingly, the *blood smear* reveals vacuoles, granules, or a combination of both in the lymphocytes of only six of nine patients and to a low degree (2%–30%) (Fig. 41).

In the *bone marrow,* the plasma cells show the most marked alterations (Fig. 42). Only a few are normal, and the majority show an abundance of lumpy, granular, and vacuolated structures, either singly or in combination. The very coarse, pink to red, and sometimes also light blue inclusions are very typical, however, and are not always circular but may be shaped almost like bricks. In the reticulum cells considerable alterations are seldom. In the osteoblasts, we observed only fine granules and no vacuoles. A fourth patient showed similar changes, but these were comparatively slight.

As for the MPSoses, the morphological characteristics of the various MLoses have been summarized schematically, and the characteristic marker cells emphasized in each disorder (Fig. 43).

**Fig. 41 a–c.** Mucolipidosis III. Blood lymphocytes.
**a** Relatively dense, fine vacuolation.
**b** Fine, reddish granules.
**c** Combination of vacuoles and granules.

**Fig. 42 a–f.** Mucolipidosis III. Bone marrow.
**a** Reticulum cell with predominantly fine, moderately dense granulation.
**b–f** Plasma cells with partly coarse, lumpy, partly granular, and partly vacuolar storage phenomena; the lumpy inclusions are of different shapes and colors.

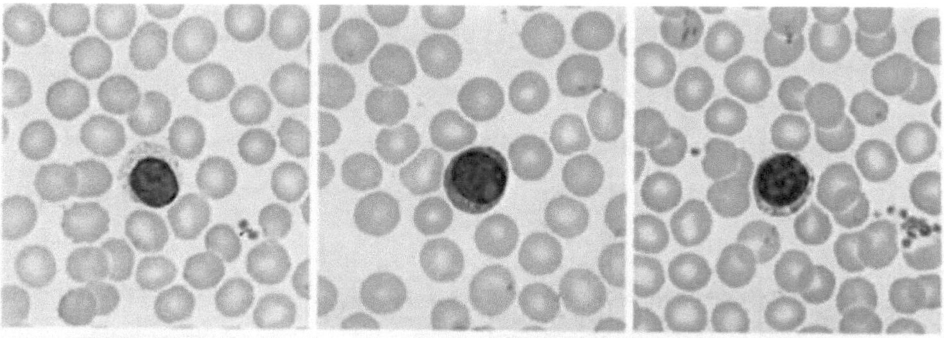
a, b
41c

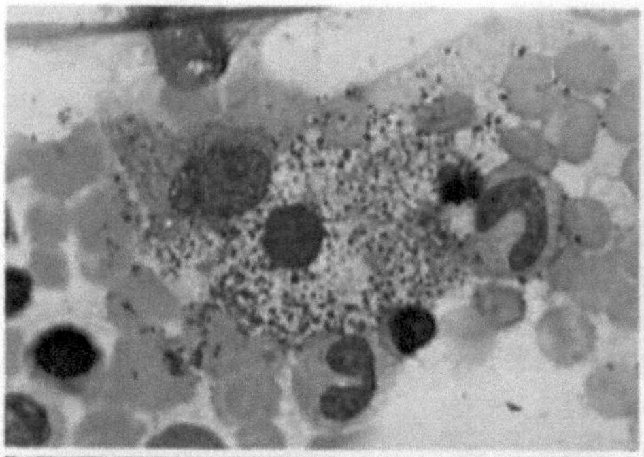
42a

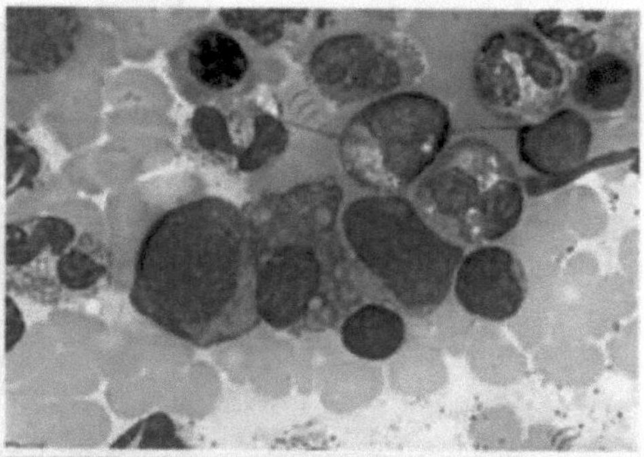
42b

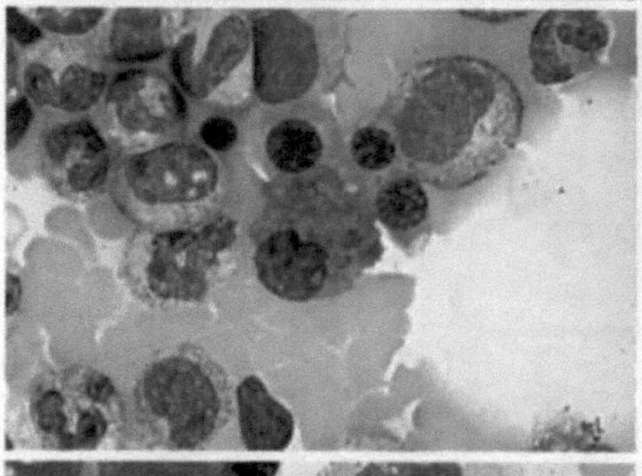
42c

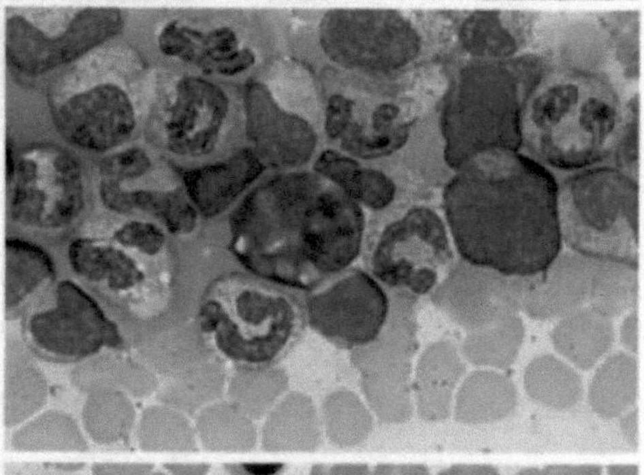
42d

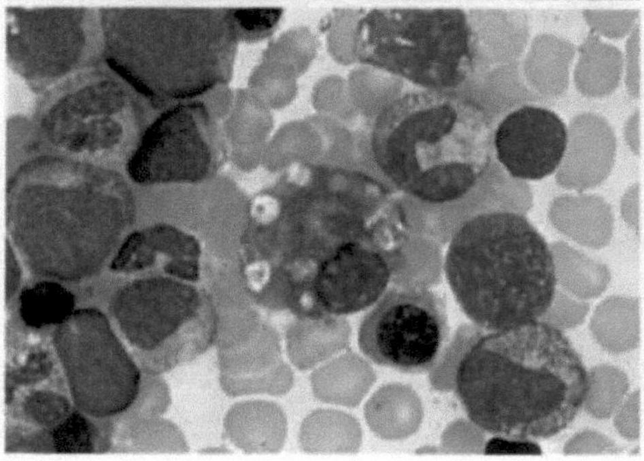
42e

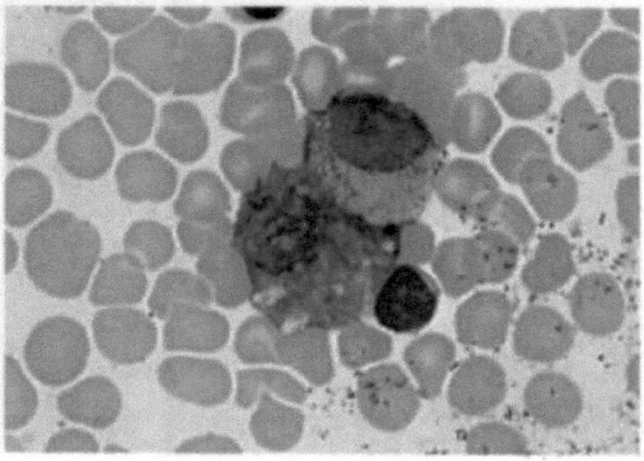
42f

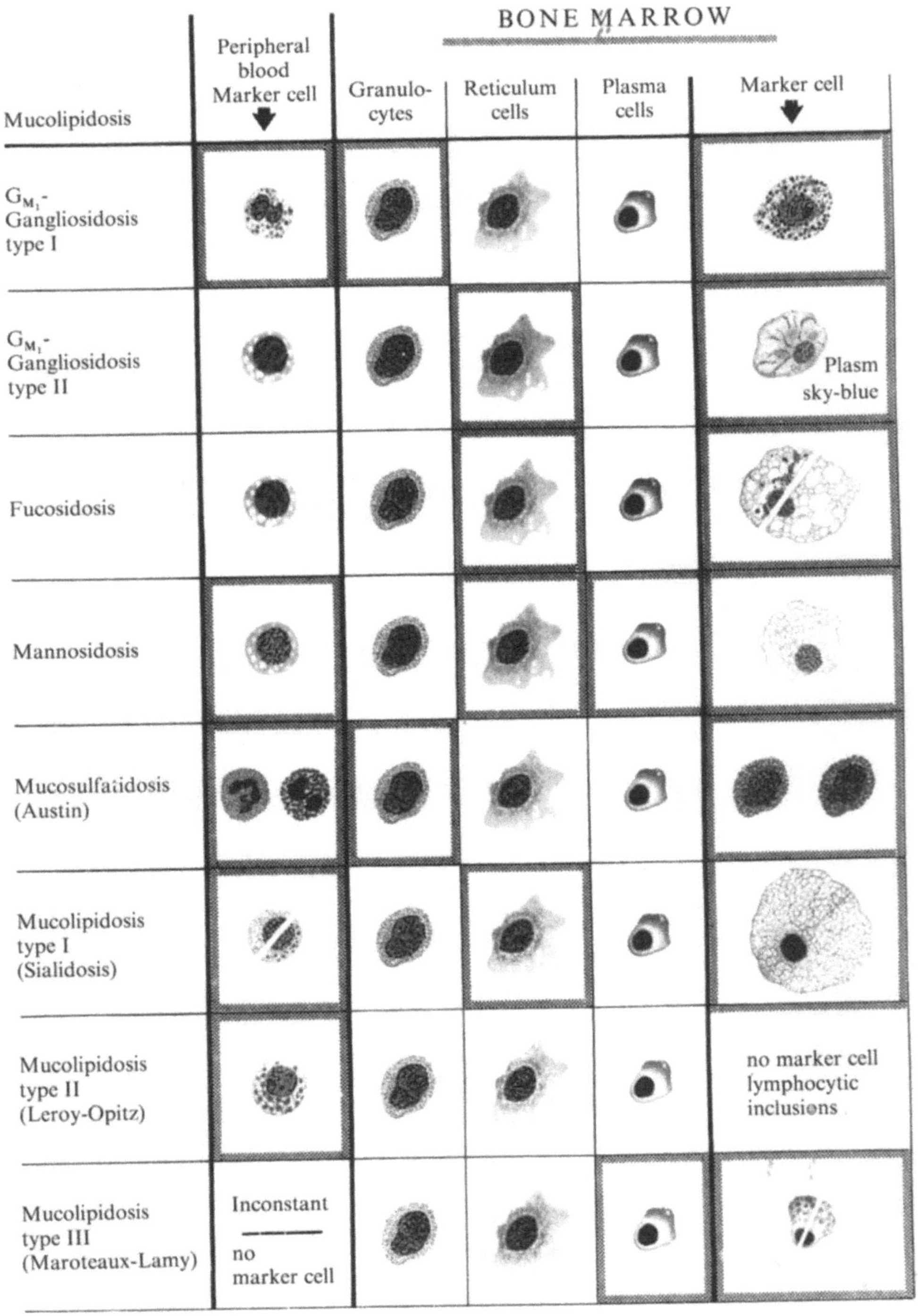


**Fig. 43.** Schematic survey of the morphologically characteristic cells (marker cells) in the mucolipidoses. Cell line derived from and marker cells bordered

# Lipidoses

In the group of lipidoses, it is the sphingolipidoses that are of prime interest. In contrast to the MPSoses and MLoses, hematomorphological changes cannot be demonstrated in all disorders for example, Krabbe's disease, and metachromatic leukodystrophy. The diseases belonging to this group are given in Table 3 (s. pp. 10–11). Apart from Fabry's disease, all sphingolipidoses have distinct clinical features, even though they are caused by a common enzyme defect. This may be due either to isoenzymes or to partial or total enzyme deficiencies. Neurological symptoms predominate, and skeletal changes play a secondary role in this group of diseases. However, hepatomegaly, splenomegaly, and ophthalmological changes can also be observed. If a splenomegaly exists, the incidence of bone marrow changes is high.

## **Niemann-Pick Disease** (Sphingomyelinase Deficiency) [37, 41]

The vacuolation of the *blood* lymphocytes reported so often in the literature could not be confirmed in the three patients we examined with Type C of the disease. However, it appears possible that changes of this type in the blood smears occur in forms characterized by total enzyme deficiencies (A and B).

In the *bone marrow,* the findings are as a rule made conspicuous by numerous round to oval reticulum cells, which are enlarged by lipid deposits. It is typical to find a mixture of fine to coarse vacuoles within a single cell (Fig. 44). These resemble the "foam cells" in $\beta$-galactosidase deficiency I, fucosidosis, and mannosidosis; however, granules are absent. Occasionally, it is possible to observe pale to medium blue tinging of the plasma instead of colorless vacuoles (Fig. 44d). Previously unreported is the more or less pronounced, fine to coarse vacuolation (30%–50%) of the plasma cells (Fig. 44f). The cell diameter is usually not enlarged.

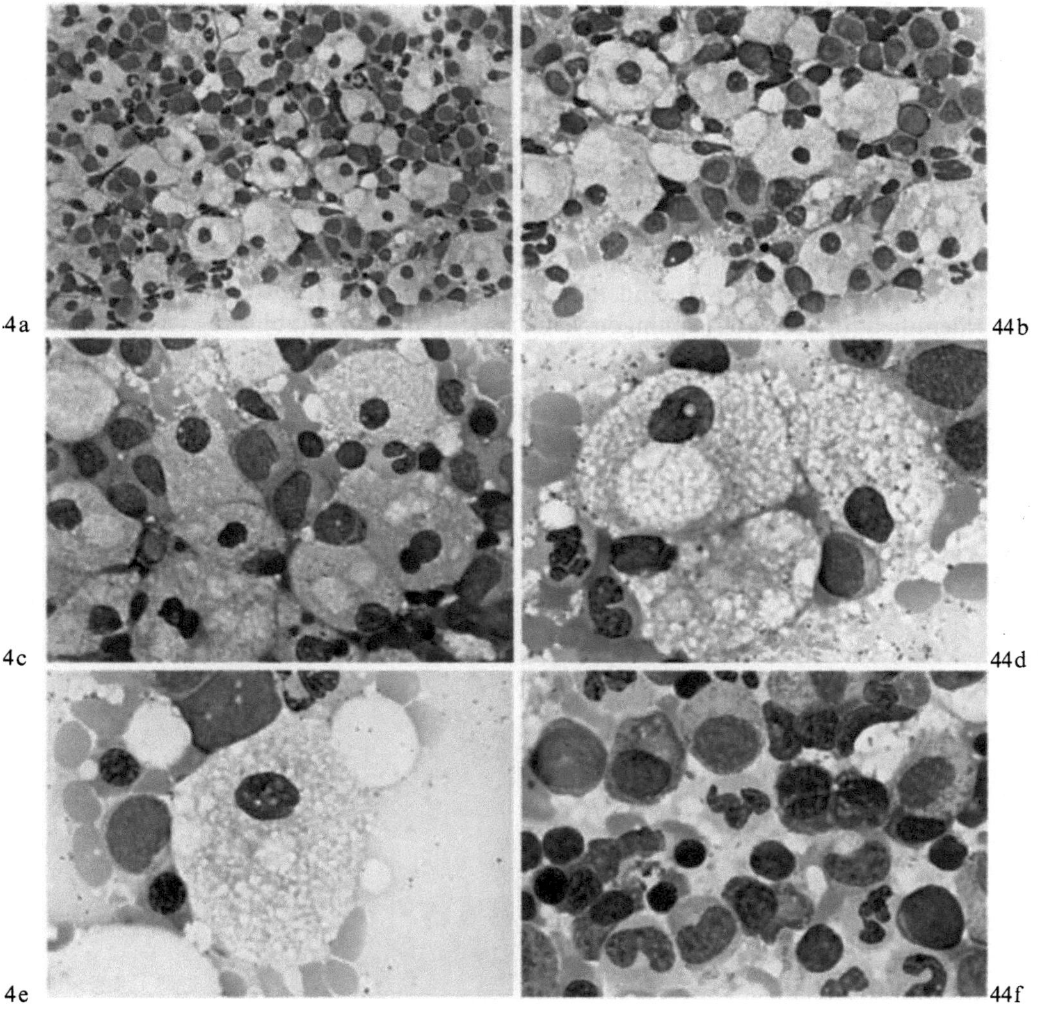


**Fig. 44a–f.** Niemann-Pick disease. Bone marrow.

**a–e** Large reticulohistiocytic storage cells, oval- to round-shaped, filled with numerous vacuoles of quite different sizes (magnification: **a** × 200, **b** × 320, **c** × 500)

**d** In part, pale blue tinging.

**f** Plasma cells with relatively fine vacuolation of varying degrees (magnification: × 500).

In **Type F,** the so-called **Sea-blue histiocyte disease** [51], we were not able to establish any changes in the peripheral *blood* of our relatively large group of seven patients either. The *marrow* is typified by phenomena similar to other forms of Niemann-Pick disease, except that the number and range of variation in the blue-tinged cells is clearly larger (Fig. 45).

We might add short comment on the problems arising with sea-blue histiocyte disease. Until 6 years ago, it was considered to be a decidedly chronic, relatively innocuous disease without neurological symptoms. Since then, the number of publications describing "Niemann-Pick-like" clinical pictures has grown (e.g., [19, 29, 62]), and the enzyme defect responsible has finally been identified (thermolabile sphingomyelinase) [53], thereby establishing its relationship to the Niemann-Pick disease.

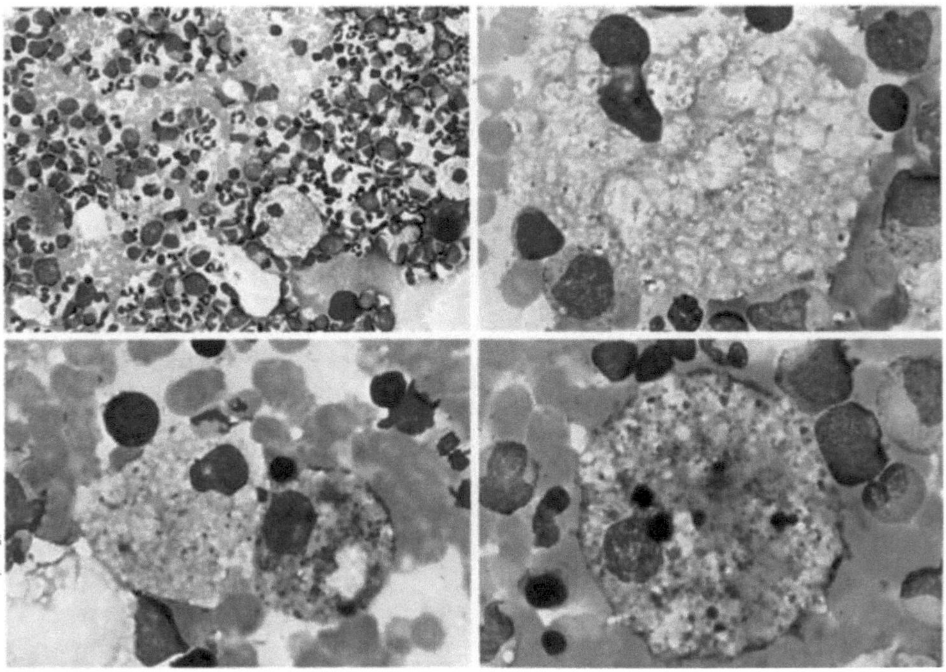

45a 45b 45c 45d

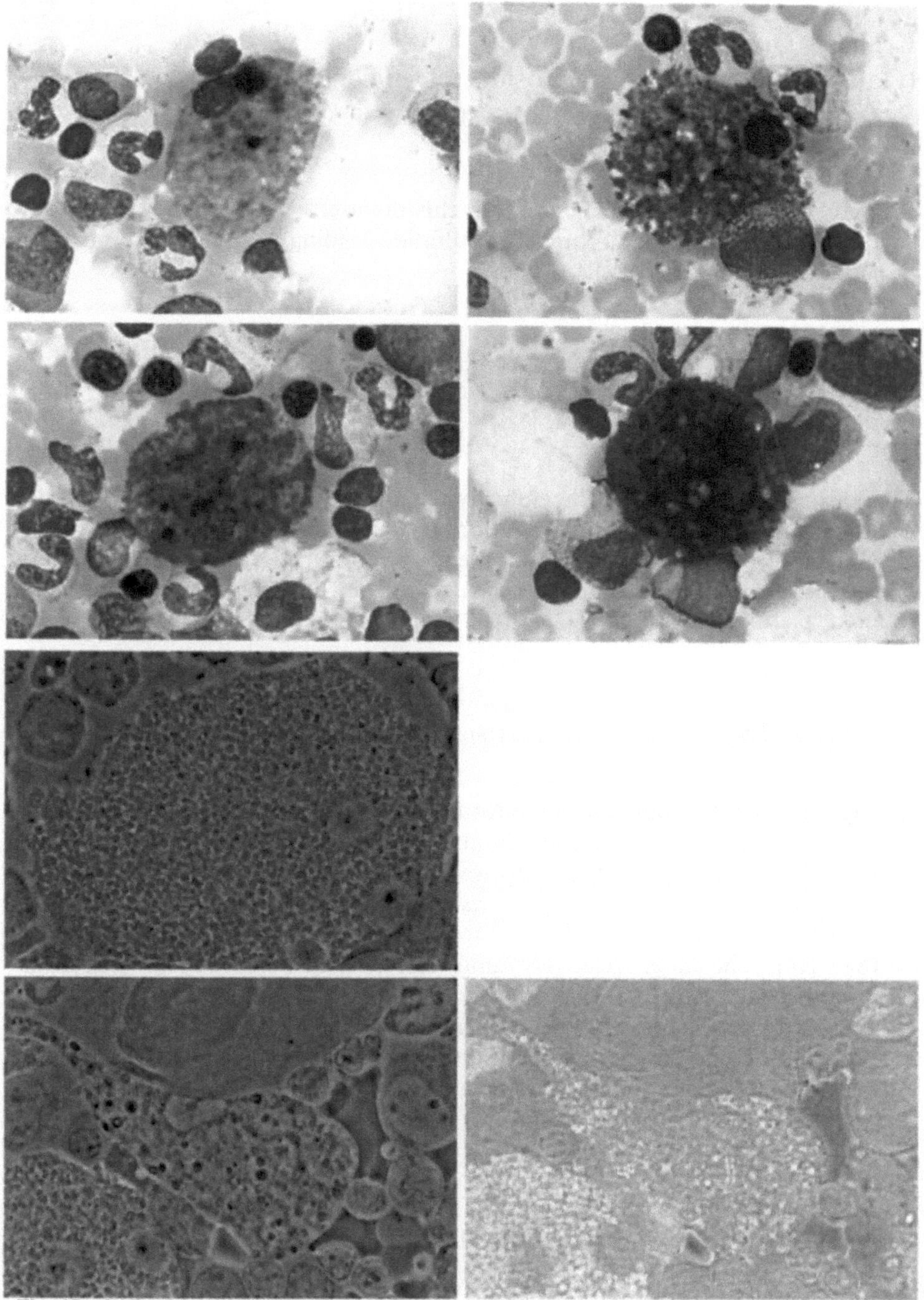

45e 45f 45g 45h 45i 45j 45k

**Fig. 45a–k.** Sea-blue histiocyte disease. Bone marrow.

**a** Several bluish storing reticulum cells scattered throughout normal marrow (magnification: ×128).

**b–h** Variants of storage cells with increasingly intense blue tinging.

**i** Large storage cell with almost homogeneous, granular structure in vital preparation (phase contrast, green filter).

**j** Storage cell in vital preparation (phase contrast, green filter).

**k** Same cell in polarized light; isolated coarse inclusions show double-refracting substances in form of so-called Maltese crosses.

## Krabbe's Disease
(Galactocerebroside-$\beta$-galactosidase Deficiency) [25]
Synonym: Globoid Cell Leukodystrophy

We have had no direct experience with this disease. Examinations carried out so far do not suggest the storage of sulfatide leading to observable changes in blood or bone marrow cells.

## Metachromatic Leukodystrophy
(Arylsulfatase A Deficiency) [18]

This disorder exhibits no storage phenomena in blood and bone marrow cells. The biochemically related mucosulfatidosis Austin (arylsulfatase A and B deficiency) has already been dealt with in the section on MLoses. The defects underlying these two diseases lead to clinically and, in particular, hematologically different pictures.

## Gaucher's Disease (Glucocerebroside-$\beta$-glucosidase Deficiency) [14]

According to current opinion, three forms of this disease occur: infantile, juvenile and adult. We were able to examine 1, 1, and 2 cases in each category respectively. From our investigations we could confirm that there are no traceable changes in the cells of the *peripheral blood.*

Gaucher's cell is the best-known storage cell and was described as early as 1882 [14]. The large, relatively uniformly shaped *bone marrow* reticulum cells show a characteristic pale gray cytoplasm which has the appearance of crumpled cigarette paper (Fig. 46). Occasionally, single vacuoles can be seen, but fibrillary structures predominate. Otherwise, similar cells are present only in isolated cases of chronic myelocytic leukemia, but of course at a much lower rate.

## Fabry's Disease ($\alpha$-Galactosidase Deficiency) [11]

Bruning [5a] described in four patients' bone marrow reticulum cells filled with fine granules which are of more or less intensive blue color. We were not able to conduct an examination ourselves.

**$G_{M1}$-gangliosidoses.** These have been dealt with in the section on MLoses (see pp. 38–43).

46a 46b 46c 46d 46e

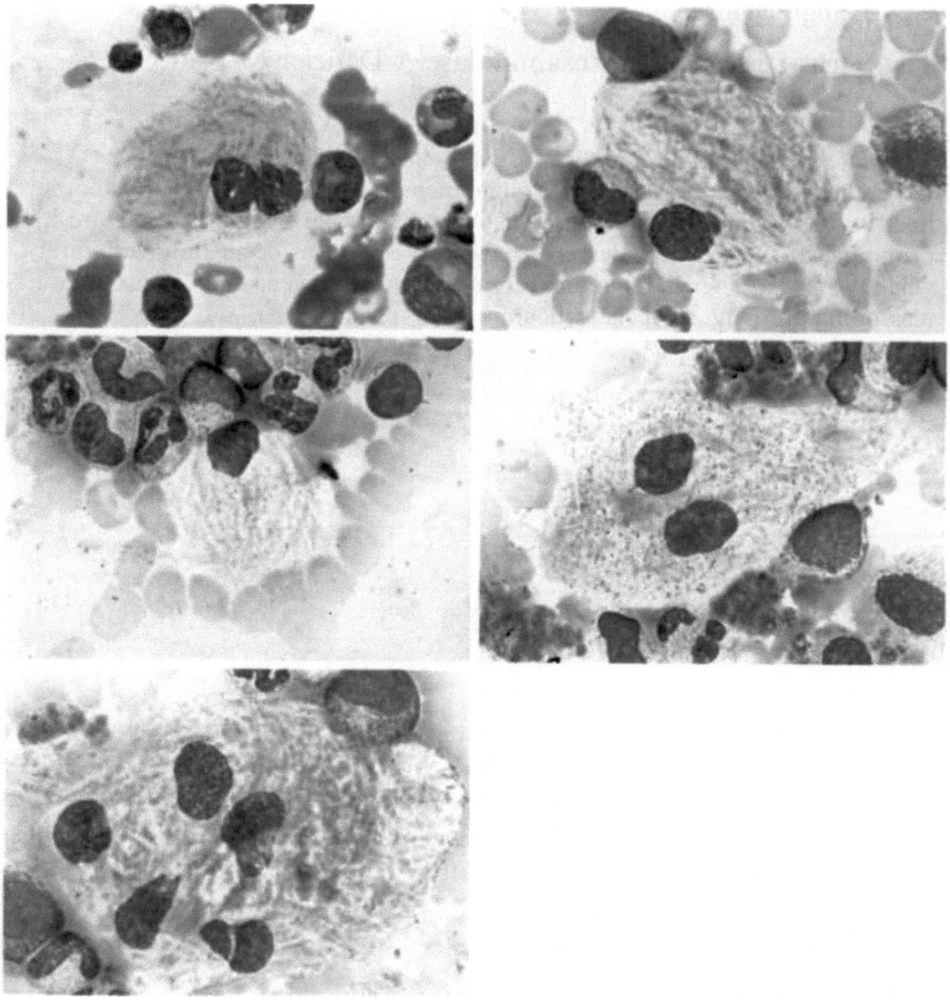

**Fig. 46a–e.** Gaucher's disease. Bone marrow. Large reticulum cells filled with storage substance; the fine, striated structures which have been compared to crumpled cigarette paper are characteristic. In **d** vary discrete granular structures are shown.

## $G_{M2}$-Gangliosidoses

### **Tay-Sachs Disease** (β-Hexosaminidase A Deficiency) [47, 59]

The *blood smear* findings are diagnostically insignificant.

In the *bone marrow,* the storage phenomena resemble those in the eosinophils in MPSoses VI and VII as well as in Austin's disease. However, they are less pronounced; i.e., exclusively red or red-violet cell forms occur only very rarely, while those characterized by a mixture of red-violet, greenish, and orange granules dominate (Fig. 47). The reticulum cells, plasma cells, and osteoblasts all remain unaltered.

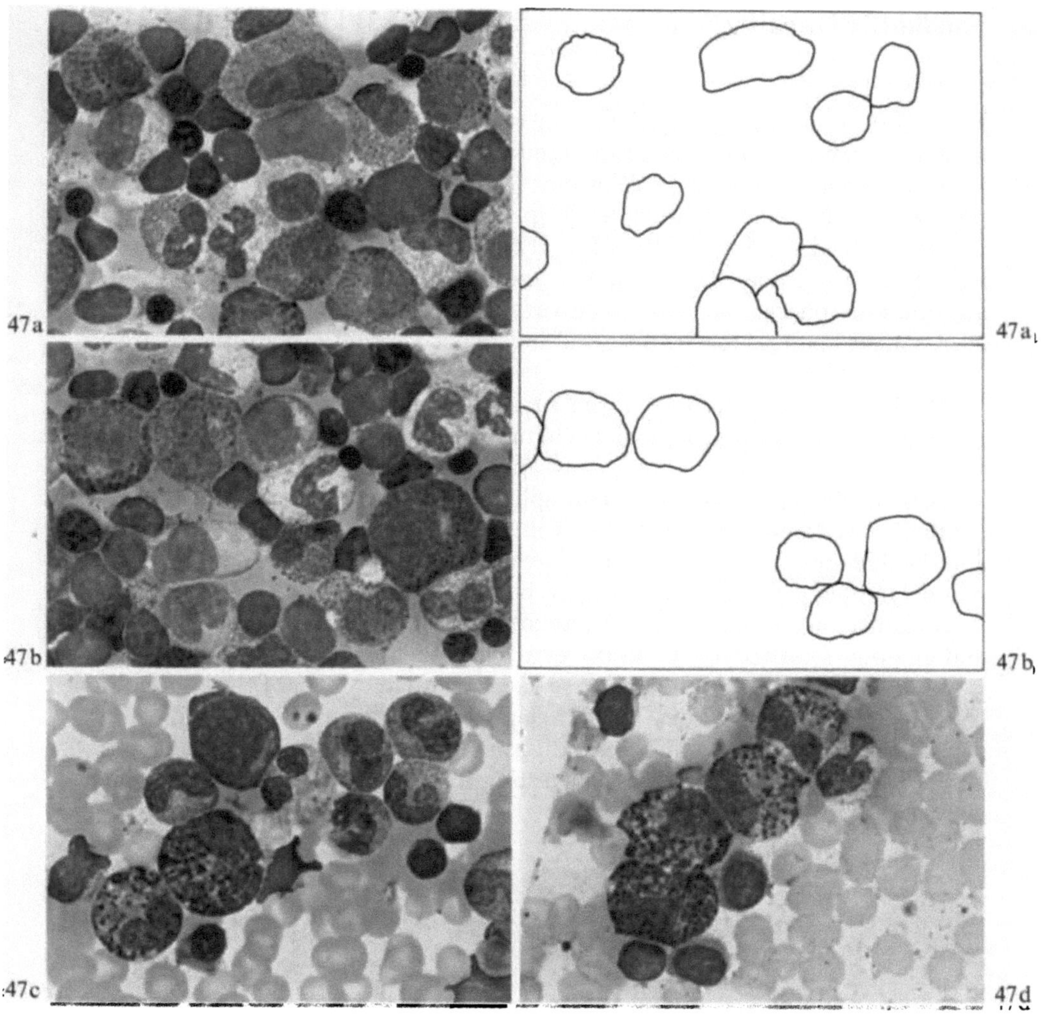


**Fig. 47a–d.** Tay-Sachs disease. Bone marrow.

**a, b** Numerous marrow eosinophils with pathologic granulation ranging from orange to greenish-gray to red-violet. On right schematic marking of eosinophils.

**c, d** Pronounced changes in eosinophils.

## **Sandhoff's Disease** (*β*-Hexosaminidase A and B Deficiency) [48]

In the *blood smear,* only isolated, unremarkable changes can be recognized, none of which have any diagnostic significance.

In the *bone marrow,* a small proportion of the plasma cells contain varying numbers of fine to coarse vacuoles (Fig. 48a–c). As a rule, the cellular diameter is not enlarged. The osteoblasts are altered, which is surprising since skeletal alterations are absent. In addition to sparse, very fine, reddish granules, there are often peripheral vacuoles which vary in size and number (Fig. 48d). However, similar changes can be observed in isolated cases of other diseases also.

We had no access to other forms of $G_{M2}$-gangliosidoses. To our knowledge, no details of hematomorphological changes have been published.

Among the lipidoses other than sphingolipidoses, only **ceroidlipofuscinosis** (Batten's disease [4]) appears to be of interest as far as frequency of occurrence and the hematomorphological aspect are concerned. In the literature, vacuolated blood lymphocytes have occasionally been mentioned (see [3, 63]). However, such changes were missing in 15 patients examined by Santavuori et al. [50] and in four reported by Gordon et al. [17]. In only one out of four cases we found a pronounced, fine to coarse vacuolation in $> 50\%$ of the lymphocytes (Fig. 49). One patient showed no storage phenomena in either the blood lymphocytes or the bone marrow. These findings are not in agreement with the apparently equivalent clinical pictures, suggesting that the basic defects are biochemically different.

48a 48b
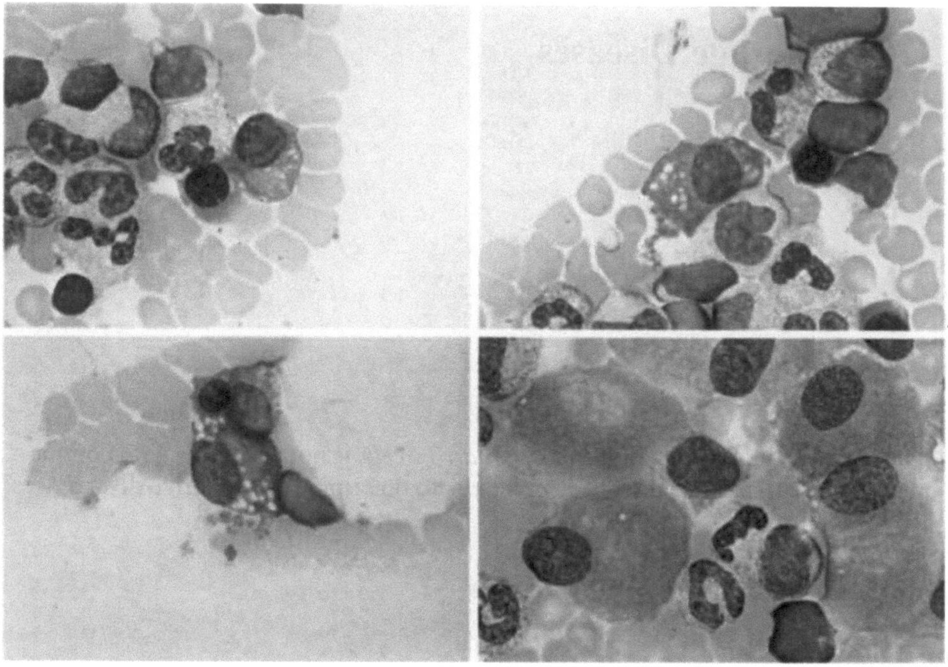
48c 48d

**Fig. 48a–d.** Sandhoff's disease. Bone marrow.

**a–c** Plasma cells with various though only moderate degrees of fine and semicoarse vacuolation.

**d** Osteoblasts with very fine, sparse, reddish granules and several, in part peripheral vacuoles.

49a 49b
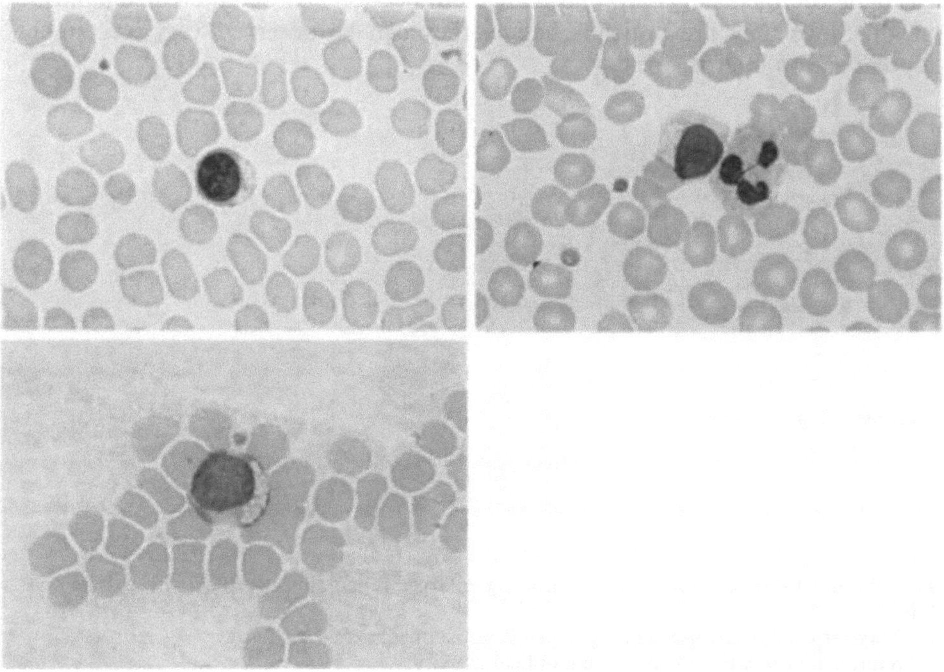
49c

**Fig. 49a–c.** Ceroidlipofuscinosis. Blood smear showing different extents of lymphocyte vacuolation.

# Other Storage Diseases

## Glycogenosis Type II

The increase of glycogen in *blood* and *marrow cells* is not verifiable with common staining methods since the problem here is to determine quantitative divergences from the norm.

## Cystinosis

Circulating *blood cells* are morphologically inconspicuous. In the *bone marrow*, there are enlarged, more or less round reticulum cells with cystine crystals (Fig. 50). The cystine deposit do not stain panoptically but are none the less easily detectable as crystals, and their identification can be taken as diagnostic proof. Since they are optically active, they can be observed very well under a polarization microscope.

50a 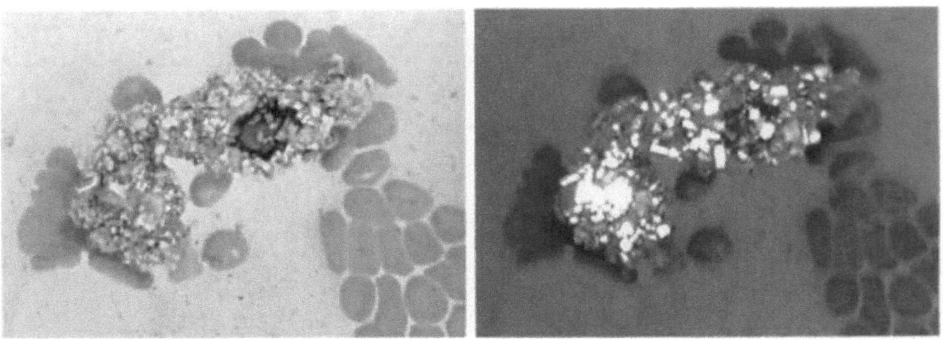 50b

**Fig. 50a, b.** Cystinosis. Bone marrow showing enlarged reticulum cells filled with cystine crystals.
**a** May-Grünwald-Giemsa staining, crystals not stained.
**b** Same cell in polarized light, strong optical activity.

# Acknowledgements

*We are indepted to the following persons and institutes for investigation material:*

E. Bühler, Basler Kinderspital
W. Burmeister, Univ.-Kinderklinik, Bonn
N. Di Ferrante, Dept. of Biochemistry, Houston
R.P. Erickson, Dept. of Pediatrics, San Francisco
P. Gibaud, Hôpital Debrousse, Lyon
B. Hagberg, Dept. of Pediatrics, Göteborg
E. Jones, Dept. of Health, Albany
W. Kosenow, Kinderklinik, Krefeld
J. Leroy, Dept. of Pediatrics, Antwerpen
R.B. Lowry, Dept. of Medical Genetics, Vancouver
P. Maroteaux, Hôpital des Enfants Malades, Paris
Irene Maumenee u. V.A. McKusick, Johns Hopkins Hospital, Baltimore
J.M. Opitz, Dept. of Genetics, Madison
R.A. Pfeiffer, Inst. für Humangenetik, Erlangen
A. Prader u. W.H. Hitzig, Kinderspital, Zürich
S.U. Rampini, Kinderspital Triemli, Zürich
E. Rupprecht, Univ.-Kinderklinik, Dresden
W.S. Sly, Childrens Hospital, St. Louis
J. Spranger, Univ.-Kinderklinik, Mainz
R.L. Summit, Dept. of Pediatrics, Memphis
H.-R. Wiedemann, Univ.-Kinderklinik, Kiel
KAV-Kinderklinik, Berlin
Univ.-Kinderklinik, Düsseldorf
Univ.-Kinderklinik, Erlangen
Univ.-Kinderklinik, Frankfurt
Neurologische Univ.-Klinik, Göttingen
Heidberg-Krankenhaus, Hamburg
Kinderklinik Rothenburgsort, Hamburg
Kinderklinik, Kassel
Kinderklinik, Kempten/Allgäu
Univ.-Kinderklinik, Kiel
Humangenetisches Institut, Münster
Univ.-Kinderklinik, Münster
Rigshospitalet, Oslo
Kinderspital, St. Gallen
Univ.-Kinderklinik, Tübingen

# References


1. ALDER A (1939) Über konstitutionell bedingte Granulationsveränderungen der Leukozyten. Dtsch Arch Klin Med 183:372–378
2. AUSTIN J, ARMSTRONG D, SHEARER L (1965) Metachromatic form of diffuse cerebral sclerosis. V. The nature and significance of low sulfatase activity. Arch Neurol 13:593–614
3. BAḠH R v., HORTLING H (1948) Blodfynd vid juvenil amaurotisk idioti. Nord Med 38:1072–1076
4. BATTEN FE (1903) Cerebral degeneration with symmetric changes in the maculae in two members of a family. Trans Ophthalmol Soc UK 23:386–390
5. BORUD O, TORP KH, DAHL T (1978) Aspartylglucosaminuria. Monogr Hum Genet 10:23–26

5a. BRUNNING, RD (1970) Morphologic alterations in nucleated blood and marrow cells in genetic disorders. Hum Pathol 1:99–124

6. DALE T (1931) Unusual forms of familial osteochondrodystrophy. Acta Radiol 12:337–358
7. DERRY DM, FACETT JS, ANDERMANN F, WOLFE LS (1968) Late infantile systemic lipidosis; major monosialogangliosidosis, delineation of two types. Neurology (Minneap) 18:340–348
8. DORFMAN A, LORINCZ AE (1957) Occurrence of urinary acid mucopolysaccharides in the Hurler syndrome. Proc Natl Acad Sci USA 43:443–446
9. DURAND P, BORRONE C, DELLA CELLA G (1966) A new mucopolysaccharide lipid storage disease? Lancet II:1313–1314
10. EICHENBERGER K (1953) Kann die Dysostose Morquio als selbständiges Krankheitsbild vom Gargoylismus abgetrennt werden? Ann Paediatr (Basel) 182:107–140
11. FABRY J (1898) Ein Beitrag zur Kenntnis der Purpura haemorrhagica nodularis (Purpura papulosa haemorrhagica Hebrae). Arch Dermatol Syphil 43:187–200
12. FRATANTONI JC, HALL CW, NEUFELD EF (1968) Hurler and Hunter syndromes: Mutual correction of the defect in cultured fibroblasts. Science 162:570–572
13. GASSER C (1950) Diskussion zum Beitrag von ALDER. Schweiz Med Wochenschr 80:1097–1098
14. GAUCHER PCE (1882) De l'épithélioma primitif de la rate. Thèse de Paris
15. GEHLER J, SEWELL AC, BECKER C, HARTMANN J, SPRANGER J (1981) Clinical and biochemical delineation of aspartyl-glucosaminuria as observed in two members of an Italian family. Helv paediat Acta 36:179–189
16. GIBAUD P, MAIRE I, GODDON R, TEYSSIER G, ZABOT MT, MANDON G (1979) Mucopolysaccharidose type VII par déficit en $\beta$-glucuronidase. Etude d'une famille. J Genet Hum 27:29–43
17. GORDON NS, MARSDEN HB, NORONHA MJ (1972) Neuronal ceroid lipofuscinosis (Batten's disease). Arch Dis Child 47:285–291
18. GREENFIELD JG (1933) Form of progressive cerebral sclerosis in infants associated with primary degeneration of interfascicular glia. Proc R Soc Med 26:690–697
19. HAGBERG B, HALTIA M, SOURANDER P, SVENNERHOLM L, VANIER M-T, LJUNGGREN C-G (1978) Neurovisceral storage disorder simulating Niemann-Pick disease. Neuropädiatrie 9:59–73
20. HANSEN HG (1972) Hematologic studies in mucopolysaccharidoses and mucolipidoses. Birth Defects 8:115–128
21. HUNTER C (1917) A rare diseae in two brothers. Proc Roy Soc Med 10:104–116

22. Hurler G (1919) Über einen Typ multipler Abartungen, vorwiegend am Skelettsystem. Z Kinderheilkd 24:220–234
23. Isenberg JN, Sharp HL (1976) Aspartylglucosaminuria: Unique biochemical and ultrastructural characteristics. Hum Pathol 7:469–481
24. Kelly TE, Thomas GH, Taylor HA, McKusick VA, Sly WS, Glaser JH, Robinow M, Luzzati L, Espiritu C, Feingold M, Bull MJ, Ashenhurst EM, Ives EJ (1975) Mucolipidosis III (pseudo-Hurler polydystrophy): Clinical and laboratory studies in a series of 12 patients. Johns Hopkins Med J 137:156–175
25. Krabbe K (1916) A new familial, infantile form of diffuse brain sclerosis. Brain 39:74–114
26. Landing BH, Silverman FN, Craig JM, Jacoby MD, Lahey ME, Chadwick DL (1964) Familial neurovisceral lipidosis. Am J Dis Child 108:503–522
27. Leroy JG, De Mars RI (1967) Mutant enzymatic and cytological phenotypes in cultured human fibroblasts. Science 157:804–806
28. Leroy JG, Spranger JW, Feingold M, Opitz JM, Crocker AC (1971) I-cell disease: A clinical picture. J Pediatr 79:360–365
29. Long RG, Lake BD, Pettit JE, Scheuer PJ, Sherlock S (1977) Adult Niemann-Pick disease. Its relationship to the syndrome of the sea-blue histiocyte. Am J Med 62:627–635
30. Maroteaux P (1973) Une nouvelle type de mucopolysaccharidose avec athétose et élimination urinaire de kératansulfate. Nouv Presse Med 2:975–979
31. Maroteaux P, Lamy M (1966) La pseudo-polydystrophie de Hurler. Presse Med 74:2889–2892
32. Maroteaux P, Leveque B, Marie J, Lamy M (1963) Une nouvelle dysostose avec élimination urinaire de chondroitinesulfate B. Presse Med 71:1849–1852
33. McKusick VA, Howell RR, Hussels IE, Neufeld EF, Stevenson RE (1972) Allelism, non-allelism and genetic compounds among the mucopolysaccharidoses. Trans Assoc Am Physicians 85:151–171
34. McKusick VA, Kaplan D, Wise D, Hanley WB, Suddarth SB, Sevick ME, Maumanee AE (1965) The genetic mucopolysaccharidoses. Medicine (Baltimore) 44:445–483
35. Morquio L (1929) Sur une forme de dystrophie osseuse familiale. Arch Méd Enfants 32:129–140
36. Neville BGR, Lake BD, Stephens R, Sanders MD (1973) A neurovisceral storage disease with vertical supranuclear ophthalmoplegia and its relationship to Niemann-Pick disease. Brain 96:97–120
37. Niemann A (1914) Ein unbekanntes Krankheitsbild. Monatsschr Kinderheilkd 79:1–10
38. O'Brien JS, Gugler E, Giedeon A, Wiessmann U, Herschkowitz N, Meier C, Leroy J (1976) Spondyloepiphyseal dysplasia, corneal clouding, normal intelligence and acid $\beta$-galactosidase deficiency. Clin Genet 9:495–504
39. Öckermann PA (1967) A generalized storage disorder resembling Hurler's syndrome. Lancet II:239–241
40. Pfaundler M v. (1919) Demonstration über einen Typus kindlicher Dysostose. MMW 66:1011
41. Pick L (1926) Der Morbus Gaucher und die ihm ähnlichen Erkrankungen. Ergeb Inn Med Kinderheilkd 29:519–627
42. Pollit RJ, Jenner FA, Merskey H (1968) Aspartylglucosaminuria. An inborn error of metabolism associated with mental defect. Lancet II:253–255
43. Rampini SU (1976) Klinik der Mukopolysaccharidosen. Enke, Stuttgart
44. Reilly WA (1941) The granules in the leukocytes in gargoylism. Am J Dis Child 62:489–491
45. Reitman ML, Varki A, Kornfeld S (1981) Fibroblasts from patients with I-cell disease and pseudo-Hurler polydystrophy are deficient in UDP-N-acetylglucosamine: Glycoprotein-N-acetylglucosaminylphosphotransferase activity. J Clin Invest 67:1574–1579
46. Royer P (1959) La cellule de Buhot et le diagnostic du gargoylisme. Sang 30:37–40
47. Sachs R (1887) On arrested cerebral development with special reference to its cortical pathology. J Nerv Ment Dis 14:541–553
48. Sandhoff R, Andreae U, Jatzkewitz H (1968) Deficient hexosaminidase activity in an

exceptional case of Tay-Sachs disease with additional storage of kidney globoside in visceral organs. Pathol Eur 3:278–285
49. Sanfilippo SJ, Podosin R, Langer L, Good RA (1963) Mental retardation associated with acid mucopolysacchariduria (heparitin sulfate type). J Pediatr 63:837–838
50. Santavuori P, Haltia M, Rapola J, Raitta C (1973) Infantile type of so-called neuronal ceroid-lipofuscinosis. Part 1. A clinical study of 15 patients. J Neurol Sci 18:257–267
51. Sawitzky A, Hyman GA, Hyman JB (1954) An unidentified reticuloendothelial cell in bone marrow and spleen: Report of two cases with histochemical studies. Blood 9:977–985
52. Scheie HG, Hambrick GW Jr, Barness LA (1962) A newly recognized forme fruste of Hurler's disease (gargoylism). Am J Ophthalmol 53:753–769
53. Schneider EL, Penchev PG, Hibbert SR, Sawitzky A, Brady RO (1978) A new form of Niemann-Pick disease characterised by temperature-labile sphingomyelinase. J Med Genet 15:370–374
54. Seringe P, Plainfosse B, Lautmann F, Lorilloux J, Calamy G, Berry JP, Watchi JM (1968) Gangliosidose généralisée du type Norman-Landing à GM1. Ann Pediatr (Paris) 44:165–184
55. Sly WS, Quinton BA, McAllister WH, Rimoin DL (1973) Beta glucuronidase deficiency: Report of clinical, radiologic and biochemical features of a new mucopolysaccharidosis. J Pediatr 82:249–257
56. Spranger J (1972) The systemic mucopolysaccharidoses. Ergeb Inn Med Kinderheilkd 32:165–265
57. Spranger J, Gehler J, Cantz M (1977) Mucolipidosis I: A sialidosis. Am J Med Genet 1:2–29
58. Spranger J, Wiedemann HR, Tolksdorf M, Graucob E, Caesar R (1968) Lipomucopolysaccharidose. Z Kinderheilkd 103:285–290
59. Tay WA (1881) Symmetrical changes in the region of the yellow spot in each eye of an infant. Trans Ophthalmol Soc UK 1:55–57
60. Undritz E (1954) Les malformations héréditaires des élements figurés du sang. Sang 25:296–324
61. Undritz E (1974) Die erblich-konstitutionellen morphologischen Anomalien der Leukocyten. In: Begemann H (ed) Blut und Blutkrankheiten, 5th edn. Springer, Berlin Heidelberg New York (Handbuch der inneren Medizin, vol 2/4)
62. Wenger DA, Barth G, Githens JH (1977) Nine cases of sphingomyelin lipidosis, a new variant in spanish-american children. Am J Dis Child 131:955–961
63. Zeman W, Dyken P (1969) Neuronal ceroid-lipofuscinosis (Batten's disease). Relationship to amaurotic familial idiocy. Pediatrics 44:570–583

# Appendix: Tables 5–8

**Table 5.** Quantitative blood cell findings in mucopolysaccharidoses (mean and range)

| Disease | Patients (n) | Neutrophils +Granules[a] | | | Eosinophils +Granules | | | Basophils | Monocytes +Granules | | Lymphocytes +Granules | | |
|---|---|---|---|---|---|---|---|---|---|---|---|---|---|
| | | fine | coarse | mixed | greenish | red-violet | mixed | Granules ↓ | fine | coarse | fine | coarse | localized |
| MPSosis I–H | 14 | 26.5<br>11.8–47.0 | 3.1<br>0–13.7 | – | 44.1<br>16.7–83.3 | 1.5<br>0–21.4 | – | 4/47 | 46.5<br>20.0–74.1 | 4.6<br>0–7.7 | 65.6<br>41.5–77.6 | 2.5<br>0–7.5 | 30.2<br>15.8–49.1 |
| MPSosis I–S | 4 | 3.5<br>0–14.0 | 12.8<br>3.0–26.2 | – | – | – | – | 0/14 | 18.7<br>5.7–30.4 | 3.6<br>0–14.3 | 22.4<br>3.7–24.0 | 1.0<br>0–2.0 | 42.9<br>0–73.2 |
| MPSosis I–H/S | 5 | 25.5<br>12.0–35.1 | – | – | 35.1<br>0–77.8 | – | – | 0/11 | 37.1<br>10.5–64.4 | 5.9<br>0–10.0 | 51.7<br>21.0–71.9 | 5.2<br>1.0–10.5 | 20.4<br>8.7–28.1 |
| MPSosis II | 24 | 22.1<br>8.6–36.0 | 0.4<br>0–4.7 | – | 36.8<br>8.3–75 | – | – | 2/57 | 35.7<br>8.0–56.4 | 3.8<br>0–12.5 | 72.2<br>52.0–90.6 | 0.7<br>0–4.0 | 31.7<br>20.0–45.7 |
| MPSosis III | 20 | 13.3<br>5.3–28.6 | – | – | 26.6<br>0–45.5 | – | – | 7/55 | 23.1<br>10.0–38.9 | 2.8<br>0–7.1 | 55.1<br>31.8–81.8 | 1.4<br>0–13.6 | 63.2<br>52.2–85.7 |
| MPSosis IV | 10 | 32.4<br>16.2–49.8 | 30.5<br>15.0–38.0 | 25.6<br>16.0–38.0 | 60.5<br>0–100 | 10.0<br>0–75.0 | – | 1/11 | 23.3<br>0–66.7 | 0.7<br>0–6.7 | 1.2<br>0–5.4 | – | 0 |
| MPSosis VI | 10 | 40.5<br>10.0–93.3 | 59.5<br>6.7–90.0 | | 1.2<br>0–10.0 | 79.0<br>30.0–100 | 19.8<br>0–66.7 | 31/49 | 52.5<br>25.0–81.2 | 44.7<br>12.4–75.0 | 33.9<br>16.2–55.2 | 4.1<br>0–8.8 | 8.0<br>0–19.4 |
| MPSosis VII | 2 | 79.6<br>69.1–90.0 | 20.4<br>10.0–30.9 | | – | 100 | – | 5/8 | 76.6<br>73.5–79.6 | 16.4<br>12.2–20.6 | 22.4<br>19.1–25.6 | 0.2<br>0–0.4 | 7.5<br>3.1–11.8 |

[a] predominantly (see also Tables 6–8)

**Table 6.** Quantitative bone marrow findings in mucopolysaccharidoses (mean and range)

| Disease | Patients (*n*) | Reticulum cells | | | | Plasma cells | | | | | Osteoblasts |
|---|---|---|---|---|---|---|---|---|---|---|---|
| | | + Granules or inclusions | | | | + Granules or inclusions | | | + Vacuoles | + Both | + Granules |
| | | fine | coarse | lumpy | polymorphic | fine | coarse | polymorphic | | | |
| MPSosis I–H | 7 | 43.2<br>29.7–59.5 | 42.8<br>32.8–50.4 | 8.3<br>1.9–16.8 | 5.6<br>1.7–12.1 | 32.4<br>25.0–43.9 | 1.5<br>0–4.2 | – | 2.6<br>0–13.1 | 4.3<br>0–30.0 | 100 |
| MPSosis I–S | 1 | 63.4 | 31.2 | 4.2 | 0.4 | 7.1 | – | – | – | – | 2/2 |
| MPSosis I–H/S | 4 | 50.8<br>37.3–65.7 | 34.2<br>26.0–40.0 | 11.6<br>2.0–25.8 | 3.5<br>1.7–5.8 | 35.0<br>25.2–45.1 | 0.8<br>0–3.2 | – | – | – | 100 |
| MPSosis II | 6 | 50.0<br>33.9–59.8 | 39.3<br>35.0–42.7 | 5.6<br>0–16.9 | 3.8<br>0–10.4 | 38.2<br>24.4–53.7 | 5.2<br>0–15.0 | 0.6<br>0–2.1 | 4.1<br>0–11.0 | 23.8<br>0–58.6 | 100 |
| MPSosis III | 12 | 85.8<br>58.1–96.8 | 9.7<br>1.8–28.8 | 0.2<br>0–1.3 | 0.7<br>0–3.8 | 32.4<br>20.6–56.0 | 16.9<br>2.7–35.5 | 24.5<br>11.4–39.3 | 0.5<br>0–3.4 | 18.8<br>0–45.2 | 100 |
| MPSosis IV | 1 | 95.0 | 2.0 | – | – | 8.0 | – | – | – | – | 10/11 |
| MPSosis VI | 1 | 72.2 | – | – | – | 31.2 | – | – | – | – | 4/6 |
| MPSosis VII | 2 | 48.0<br>34.1–61.8 | – | – | – | 13.0<br>9.4–16.5 | – | – | 16.5<br>0–32.9 | 4.2<br>2.5–5.9 | 7/7 |

**Table 7.** Quantitative blood cell findings in mucolipidoses (mean and range)

| Disease | Patients (*n*) | Neutrophils | Eosinophils | | | |
|---|---|---|---|---|---|---|
| | | +Granules | +Granules | | Granules diminished | |
| | | | greenish | red-violet mixed | ↓ | ↓↓ |
| β-Galactosidase deficiency I | 3 | – | 5.1<br>3.2–12.0 | – | 39.0<br>29.0–44.0 | 55.9<br>44.0–67.8 |
| β-Galactosidase deficiency II and III | 3 | – | 25.3<br>0–45.8 | – | 54.2<br>12.5–100 | – |
| Fucosidosis | 1 | 7.0 | 7.9 | – | 27.6 | – |
| Mannosidosis | 15 | 1.0<br>0–3.2 | 9.9<br>0–28.6 | – | 59.1<br>28.6–100 | 3.7<br>0–40.0 |
| Aspartylglucosaminuria | 2 | 3.5<br>2.0–5.0 | 11.8<br>0–23.5 | – | – | – |
| Mucosulfatidosis | 5 | 100.0 | – | 100.0 | – | – |
| Mucolipidosis I | 2 | 5.8<br>4.0–7.0 | – | – | 3/3 | – |
| Mucolipidosis II | 5 | 0.6<br>0–2.0 | 27.4<br>6.7–62.8 | – | – | – |
| Mucolipidosis III | 9 | 0.7<br>0–5.9 | 6.3<br>0–27.2 | – | – | – |

| Monocytes | | | Lymphocytes | | | | | |
|---|---|---|---|---|---|---|---|---|
| +Granules | +Vacuoles | +Both | +Vacuoles | | +Granules | +Both | +Lumps | Pathologic total |
| | | | fine | coarse | | | | |
| 1.1<br>0–3.3 | 43.0<br>33.3–52.5 | 30.0<br>16.7–53.3 | 59.8<br>51.0–68.8 | 28.6<br>18.4–33.0 | 0.6<br>0.5–0.8 | 1.0<br>0.8–1.5 | – | 90.0<br>87.5–94.7 |
| 1.1<br>0–3.3 | 47.6<br>40.0–61.9 | 6.7<br>0–20.0 | 38.6<br>32.0–49.6 | 12.0<br>1.0–33.8 | 1.0<br>0–1.8 | 0.5<br>0–1.4 | – | 52.1<br>38.6–89.2 |
| 1.8 | 27.9 | – | 20.8 | 0.4 | 0.8 | – | – | 22.0 |
| 11.5<br>0–25.0 | 18.4<br>0–50.0 | 21.3<br>0–60.8 | 48.3<br>21.6–71.0 | 10.8<br>0–42.4 | 1.4<br>0–3.2 | 2.3<br>0–4.2 | – | 62.8<br>33.0–87.6 |
| – | 32.1<br>27.7–36.4 | 2.8<br>0–5.5 | 26.0<br>18.4–33.6 | 0.4<br>0–0.8 | 0.2<br>0–0.4 | – | – | 26.6<br>19.2–34.0 |
| 94.9<br>90.5–100 | – | – | – | – | 52.8<br>29.6–73.5 | – | – | 52.8<br>29.6–73.5 |
| – | 23.8<br>17.6–28.8 | – | 15.1<br>13.0–17.0 | 7.4<br>4.8–12.0 | 0.4<br>0–0.8 | – | – | 22.9<br>20.8–29.0 |
| 2.2<br>0–10.8 | 1.6<br>0–8.0 | – | 1.7<br>0–3.0 | 1.0<br>0–2.4 | 10.7<br>4.3–16.0 | 14.1<br>6.7–18.8 | 4.4<br>0.8–10.7 | 31.9<br>18.5–39.2 |
| 1.0<br>0–9.1 | 1.4<br>0–6.0 | – | 1.7<br>0–4.4 | 0.2<br>0–1.1 | 3.5<br>0–17.6 | 2.6<br>0–7.6 | – | 8.0<br>0–30.0 |

**Table 8.** Quantitative bone marrow findings in mucolipidoses (mean and range)

| | Patients (n) | Reticulum cells | | | | | | |
|---|---|---|---|---|---|---|---|---|
| | | + Vacuoles | | | + Granules | | + Both | Special cells |
| | | fine | coarse | mixed | fine | coarse | | |
| β-Galactosidase deficiency I | 3 | 12.3<br>2.3–27.6 | 16.4<br>11.4–19.2 | 22.0<br>15.9–29.8 | 4.2<br>0–9.1 | 3.0<br>0–9.1 | 40.6<br>29.2–52.2 | – |
| β-Galactosidase deficiency II and III | 5 | 6.4<br>3.6–9.7 | – | – | 20.3<br>3.2–38.7 | 3.5<br>0.7–8.1 | 2.8<br>0–8.3 | „Sky-blue"<br>63.5<br>37.1–85.3 |
| Fucosidosis | 1 | 22.9 | 14.2 | 7.0 | 19.6 | 2.6 | 18.0 | – |
| Mannosidosis | 6 | 9.0<br>4.6–13.1 | 5.7<br>2.0–10.7 | 5.7<br>2.4–11.4 | 5.6<br>0–14.3 | – | 63.2<br>44.5–76.2 | – |
| Mucosulfatidosis | 2 | – | – | – | 68.9<br>62.2–75.5 | 28.1<br>20.4–35.7 | – | – |
| Mucolipidosis I | 2 | 68.0<br>64.0–72.0 | 13.5<br>13.0–14.0 | 2.5<br>1.0–4.0 | 0.5<br>0–1.0 | – | 15.5<br>13.0–18.0 | – |
| Mucolipidosis II | 2 | 30.0<br>22.0–38.0 | 3.0<br>0–6.0 | 2.0<br>0–4.0 | 11.5<br>11.0–12.0 | 0.5<br>0–1.0 | 35.0<br>10.0–60.0 | – |
| Mucolipidosis III | 3 | 10.0<br>0–30.0 | – | – | 2.0<br>0–6.0 | – | – | – |

| asma cells | | | | | Osteoblasts | | |
|---|---|---|---|---|---|---|---|
| Vacuoles | | + Granules | | + Both | + Vacuoles | + Granules | + Both |
| ne | coarse | fine | coarse | | | | |
| .5<br>.1–27.8 | 23.1<br>0–41.7 | 0.9<br>0–2.8 | – | 1.9<br>0–5.6 | – | 11.0<br>0–33.0 | 89.0<br>75–100 |
| .7<br>.8–22.2 | 3.4<br>0–5.8 | 2.5<br>0–5.6 | – | – | 12.2<br>0–57.1 | 35.2<br>14.3–58.8 | 49.4<br>28.6–62.5 |
| .2 | – | – | – | – | Osteoblasts not detected | | |
| .0<br>.8–39.1 | 58.7<br>33.2–78.3 | 0.5<br>0–1.3 | – | 0.4<br>0–1.2 | – | 20.8<br>0–100 | 79.2<br>0–100 |
| | – | 52.7<br>(16.1 = also polymorphic)<br>45.1–60.2 | 19.9<br><br>5.6–34.2 | 2.8<br><br>1.0–4.6 | – | 91.5<br><br>83.3–100 | – |
| .4<br>.5–3.2 | 3.9<br>3.0–4.8 | 1.6<br>1.5–1.6 | – | – | – | – | 100 |
| .0<br><br>.7–13.3 | 8.4<br><br>6.7–10.0 | 13.7<br><br>10.0–17.3 | 30.9<br>(24.9 = also lumpy)<br>18.4–43.4 | 23.6<br><br>20.0–27.2 | – | – | 100 |
| .8<br><br>.0–11.8 | 13.0<br><br>6.3–23.8 | 13.0<br><br>5.0–17.7 | 27.5<br>(33.6 = also lumpy)<br>23.7–33.4 | 30.9<br><br>22.2–41.5 | – | 6/6 | – |

# Subject Index